The Easy Guide to OSCEs for Communication Skills

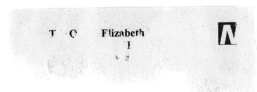

The Easy Guide to OSCEs for Communication Skills

MUHAMMED AKUNJEE
GP Principal

NAZMUL AKUNJEE
GP Registrar

SHOAIB SIDDIQUI
Specialist Medical Training

and

ALI SAMEER MALLICK
Specialist Surgical Training

Foreword by
JOHN S ROHAN

Radcliffe Publishing
Oxford • New York

Radcliffe Publishing Ltd
18 Marcham Road
Abingdon
Oxon OX14 1AA
United Kingdom

www.radcliffe-oxford.com

Electronic catalogue and worldwide online ordering facility.

British Library Cataloguing in Publication Data

A catalogue record for this book is available from the British Library.

ISBN-13: 978 184619 338 5

The paper used for the text pages of this book
is FSC certified. FSC (The Forest Stewardship
Council) is an international network to promote
responsible management of the world's forests.

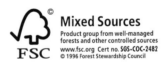

Mixed Sources
Product group from well-managed
forests and other controlled sources
www.fsc.org Cert no. SGS-COC-2482
© 1996 Forest Stewardship Council

Typeset by Pindar NZ, Auckland, New Zealand
Printed and bound by TJI Digital, Padstow, Cornwall, UK

Contents

Preface

Communication skills are an essential component of modern-day medicine. Doctors continually engage with patients to alleviate their difficulties and they have to deal with a whole host of problems. Through effective communication skills, a doctor will be able to gain a detailed insight into the patient's illness and its context, thereby making the correct diagnosis and subsequently treating them.

It is now a recognised fact that communication plays a pivotal role in the doctor–patient relationship. For this reason, medical schools have begun to focus on communication skills from the very moment the student begins their studies. Despite the increased exposure to communication-skill teaching, many students still find the vernacular and medical jargon mind-boggling. Many of the available books and literature on communication skills are targeted at senior doctors and researchers who have had many years of patient exposure. As a result, the content of such texts may appear irrelevant and far too time-consuming for the student and newly qualified doctor to digest.

For this reason, we have written *The Easy Guide to OSCEs for Communication Skills* to lighten the load of the already over-burdened medical student. With this book, we aim to simplify communication skills by breaking down some of its theories and concepts, whilst illustrating them through practical role plays. This book covers a wide selection of common dilemmas that students and doctors alike would be expected to handle competently, both in the clinical and examination settings. It also tackles some of the more challenging and increasingly familiar scenarios, such as cross-cultural sensitivities, communicating with a patient whose first language is not English, and dealing with patients' complaints about their treatment.

We hope that this book, the final volume in the *Easy Guide to OSCEs* series, will replicate some of the successes of the previous two books and go on to make communication skills interesting and accessible to its readers.

Muhammed Akunjee
Nazmul Akunjee
Shoaib Siddiqui
Ali Sameer Mallick
May 2010

Foreword

Medicine is all about obtaining a history, undertaking an examination, recommending appropriate investigations and designing a management plan for our patients. Our mentors and teachers have taught us the basis of medicine and equipped us with the skills to diagnose and treat illnesses. However, in contemporary medical practice, these are insufficient to make a well-rounded clinician.

Although newly qualified doctors have a wide range of practical skills, it is disappointing to find that very few of them have been instilled with the necessary listening, communication and self-reflection skills needed to ease the patient's journey.

This book seeks to address this issue head on and includes chapters on the consultation, communicating with colleagues, and dealing with mistakes and complaints – crucial areas for doctors to further develop their skills. It is written in a clear and refreshing style that helps to demystify this vast and complex topic.

The book will undoubtedly aid confidence building in communication and provide a superb framework to tackle scenarios encountered in examinations as well as clinical practice. It will be a vital revision aid for under- and postgraduate exams, as well as a valuable reference tool for doctors wishing to improve their communication skills as part of their everyday practice.

Dr John S Rohan MBBCh FRCGP
GP Partner, Trainer, GP Appraiser and
Collaborative Clinical Lead, Haringey PCT
Former GPVTS Course Organiser
May 2010

About the authors

Muhammed Akunjee MBBS MRCGP PgCert (Diabetes) PgCert (MedEd)
Muhammed Akunjee is currently a GP Principal in North London and works as Mental Health Lead for the South-East Collaborative for the local PCT. He qualified from Guy's, King's and St Thomas' Medical School in 2002 and completed his MRCGP, gaining an overall distinction, in 2006. During this time he was also awarded first prize for the Roche/RCGP Registrar award.

He completed a Postgraduate Certificate in Medical Education at the University of Dundee and, more recently, a Certificate in Diabetes at Warwick University. He is involved in medical student teaching and is currently a clinical-skills tutor at a London university. He is an avid medical writer and has had a number of articles published in peer-review publications.

Nazmul Akunjee MBBS
Nazmul Akunjee is currently engaged in his GP vocational training as a GP Registrar. He qualified from Guy's, King's and St Thomas' Medical School in 2005 and is currently actively engaged in teaching medical students and preparing them for their exams. He has also published a number of articles related to examination skills in OSCEs.

Nazmul Akunjee and Muhammed Akunjee are both authors of *The Easy Guide to OSCEs for Final Year Medical Students*, which was Commended in the 2008 BMA Book Awards. With the assistance of Shoaib Siddiqui, *The Easy Guide to OSCEs for Specialties* was Highly Commended in the 2009 BMA Book Awards.

Shoaib Siddiqui MBBS BSc
Shoaib Siddiqui is currently a core medical trainee at Barts and the London NHS Trust. He graduated from King's College London in 2007 and has a BSc in Physiology with Basic Sciences. He is actively involved in teaching medical students of all years.

Ali Sameer Mallick MBBS
Sameer Mallick graduated from King's College London in 2007. After completing his Foundation Year training in the Kent, Surrey and Sussex Deanery, Sameer successfully secured an Academic Clinical Fellowship in ENT. He is currently working at the Queen's Medical Centre in Nottingham.

CHAPTER 1

Introduction and basic consultation skills

Human beings are social, interactive creatures that are distinguished from animals due to their ability to reason, rationalise and reflect upon their surroundings. They form intricate social networks using language and emotion as a basis to these relationships. These networks grow to formulate communities and complex societies which function in a uniform and cohesive manner. Being able to communicate, therefore, is an essential part of the human makeup.

As doctors, we have been given a privileged role in society to cater for the health needs of the population. Patients from all walks of life and differing backgrounds present themselves to us in search of help, advice and solutions to their medical and social problems. Being able to elicit a patient's complaints and arrive at a diagnosis will require effective and efficient communication skills. These skills will also be crucial in laying down the foundation for a successful doctor–patient relationship.

In recent times, more emphasis has been placed on the teaching of good communication skills at an earlier stage in medical training. This is because there is a wealth of evidence that has linked good communication with positive health outcomes such as improved symptom resolution, reduced exacerbation of chronic illnesses and medication concordance. In addition, good communication has been shown to increase patient satisfaction, which in turn leads to a reduction in complaints and litigious proceedings.

Whilst it is difficult to *quantify* good communication, its qualities comprise a set of learnable skills and techniques that can be used during any consultation. This chapter aims to define what good communication is and how one may utilise it appropriately in the doctor–patient relationship.

DOCTOR–PATIENT CONSULTATION

The doctor–patient relationship is the medium through which the doctor is able to elicit details about the patient's problem. It is based upon key principles that include mutual trust, respect and honesty. The stronger the relationship, the more likely it is for the patient to divulge important personal information that will aid the doctor's ability to diagnose.

In days gone by, health professionals employed a consultation model that was largely doctor-centred and paternalistic. What this meant was that the doctor would ask a battery of closed questions to elicit precise responses from the patient before formulating a diagnosis. Much of the communication was unilateral, with the patient playing a limited role in the decision-making process. It was thought that the doctor knew better and the patient was expected to simply adhere religiously to their advice. The patient's own ideas about their health were disregarded and their understanding overlooked. As a result, the patient often felt disengaged from the process and would be more likely to default on the advice given. With the passage of time, it has been recognised that such a model is ineffective and is now out of vogue.

A patient-centred approach, on the other hand, was found to yield improved patient satisfaction and compliance with advice and treatment. A patient-centred model is one in which the consultation is focused primarily around the patient's needs and their concerns. The doctor uses open questions as well as verbal and non-verbal forms of communication to engage the patient and permit them to express themselves freely. Their ideas about their condition and any allied concerns are actively sought. The patient is seen to be an equal partner in the consultation process, whose opinion is valued and respected.

Communication skills

Communication is the art of conveying information from one individual to another. Most people understand communication to be simply the use of language. Whilst superficially this may be the case, good communication is in fact more complicated than this. Communication is a dynamic, two-way process that involves speaking, listening and observing. The speaking aspect corresponds to verbal communication, whereas listening and observing falls under non-verbal communication. Both forms of communication when used in conjunction with one another allows you to gain a comprehensive picture about the patient and their health needs.

Verbal communication

Verbal communication, as the name suggests, is the form of communication that is orally transmitted. It is communication that centres around words, speech and language. Through its use, thoughts and ideas can be exchanged between individuals.

Although it is often thought that the *content* of what is being said is the most important, research suggests that the effectiveness of communication hinges around *how it is said*. Factors such as the tone of voice, speed of delivery and the complexity of the information may affect the impact of what is being said.

Speed and tone of voice

The vocal tone and speed by which you communicate may alter the meaning and importance of what is being said. Speaking hastily and in a high-pitched tone may be interpreted as being anxious and nervous. Conversely, speaking slowly and in a low-pitched tone may be seen as being empathic or, in other circumstances, suggestive that something important is about to be discussed.

Jargon

Much time is spent in medical school learning complex new terminologies and vernacular. Doctors use these terms so frequently when communicating with one another that it may seem, to the untrained ear, as if they are conversing in a foreign language. These terms are often so entrenched in the doctors' vocabulary that they may unwittingly assume that the patient and the general public are equally *au fait* with them. The reality is that the vast majority of the public have limited degrees of understanding about such words and will rarely volunteer their ignorance.

If the doctor uses medical jargon when communicating with the patient, it may cause them to feel anxious, confused and ill-informed. It may also lead to misinformation and misunderstandings, potentially putting the patient at risk of harm.

To prevent this from happening, doctors should try to steer away from using medical jargon. Time should be spent simplifying the content of what you wish to tell the patient, to ensure that it is understood correctly. For example, instead of telling a patient that they require a laparoscopic cholecystectomy, it may be better to use words such as 'gallbladder' and 'keyhole surgery'.

Bite-size information and pausing

The *amount* of information you impart to the patient may also affect their ability to digest its content. The patient is likely to be anxious and tense, especially if they are awaiting important test results. If, when explaining a diagnosis to the patient, you were to overload them with excessive information and unnecessary detail, it is more than likely that they will be left bamboozled. Patients may then leave the consultation frustrated and more confused than when they initially presented.

A better approach would be to organise the information into small segments that can be disclosed to the patient at a slower pace. It may also be beneficial to intersperse the information with short pauses that will afford the patient time to comprehend the points you are trying to make.

Pauses are equally as helpful to the doctor as to the patient. They give the doctor a brief moment to organise their thoughts before continuing. They also allow time to observe the patient for any emotional responses or cues they may display. Be careful in prolonging a pause unnecessarily or using them too often, as this may hold the suspense for too long and cause annoyance and impatience in the patient.

Non-verbal communication

Non-verbal forms of communication relate to communication that takes place between individuals without the use of language. Studies have shown that when communicating information, verbal communication carries only about 40% of the message whilst non-verbal communication makes up for the remaining 60%. This indicates that communication is not only about what you say but rather how you go about saying it.

Non-verbal communication utilises your observation skills to monitor facial expressions, gestures and body language. It also requires active listening skills to take on board and consider what the patient is actually saying.

Eye contact

Making eye contact is an essential aspect of non-verbal communication. It simply involves maintaining an active focus of one person's gaze upon another. People often probe the eyes to get telltale signs of truthfulness, warmth, attraction, anger or sadness. Doctors should try to make good eye contact with their patients as this will inspire confidence and demonstrate that you are actively interested in what they are saying. Failure to do so may make you appear rude and discourteous and leave the patient feeling ignored.

Try not to make prolonged eye contact or stare out the patient as this may be interpreted as being domineering and aggressive. In some cultures, particularly between opposite genders, eye contact may be frowned upon. Take into account cultural sensitivities and make allowances accordingly. If, during the consultation, the patient fails to maintain good eye contact, this may be a cue that something is amiss. They could be depressed, anxious or simply attempting to conceal some information from you.

Facial expression

A person's face can be a mirror that reflects their innermost feelings. Through facial expressions emotions, such as fear, happiness, anger, excitement or frustration, may be revealed. By observing the patient's face the doctor may also gauge the patient's degree of engagement, as well as pick up any cues indicating confusion or concern. For example, if, when you are explaining a diagnosis, you notice that the patient's facial expressions appear blank or confused, it is more than likely they have lost the thread of the discussion. On the other hand, if you notice that they are frowning or grimacing, this may suggest that they are upset with something you have said.

Posture

How a patient holds their posture can give you some insight as to how they are feeling. A patient sitting cross-armed and cross-legged, slouching in the chair may be uninterested and disengaged. In contrast, a patient who adopts an open posture with arms and legs uncrossed, and slightly leant forward is probably relaxed and attentive to what you are saying. As a doctor, you should try to adopt an open posture throughout the consultation as this conveys feelings of warmth and appears welcoming to the patient.

Touch

Touch is a form of non-verbal communication that can transmit feelings of safety, warmth and compassion. It is a very difficult skill to employ effectively during the consultation as it is easily misinterpreted. In today's litigious and culturally diverse society, touch probably plays less of a role than in the past. It may still be used, particularly when breaking bad news, as a way to console the patient and express empathy. It is often a spontaneous gesture that occurs at the spur of the moment. However, it is important that both parties are comfortable with this reaction for it to be successful and achieve its aim.

Active listening

When two people are conversing, at any one time one person will be talking whilst the other is listening. However, just because a person remains silent this does not mean that they are necessarily paying attention to what is being said. As a doctor, you should try to demonstrate to the patient that you are interested in what they are saying by actively listening to them. This can be done by either nodding your head or through verbal encouragement such as saying, 'Yes', 'Hmm', or 'OK, go on'.

Another way to demonstrate this is to reflect back key terms and words that the patient has used in conversation. This will instil confidence in the patient that you are paying attention and have understood what they have said.

BARRIERS TO LISTENING

Remaining attentive to what the patient is saying may at times be an arduous process. There are a number of potential pitfalls that you may unconsciously fall into in order to expedite this. However, these pitfalls may act as a barrier to active and effective listening and should be avoided. Some examples include:

Assuming – this is when the doctor attempts to second-guess the real purpose of the patient's attendance rather than listening to what the patient is saying. For example, a frequent attendee to your practice may present with back pain and you assume that their real agenda is to obtain a sick note.

Associating – this is when the doctor associates the patient's symptoms with those of another patient they have managed in the past. For example, a young builder presents with chest pain. You may hastily diagnose them with musculo-skeletal pain and forget to enquire about the patient's recent travel abroad (risk factor for pulmonary embolism).

Cherry-picking – this is when the doctor selectively listens out for parts of the history that conform to the working diagnosis and ignores everything else. For example, a doctor diagnosing a banker with tension headaches while ignoring their complaints that their headache worsens on walking, and is associated with photophobia and early morning vomiting (possibly symptomatic of a cerebral space-occupying lesion).

Rehearsing – this is when the doctor is more concerned about how to phrase the next question rather than listening to the patient's response to the last question. For example, a medical student may be preoccupied with phrasing their next question about social history without actually listening to the patient's response about their drug allergies.

Prejudicing – this is when a doctor judges a patient because of their background, ethnicity, gender or age. An example of this would be a doctor meeting an elderly patient for the first time and assuming that they are cognitively impaired.

Verbal and non-verbal cues

Patients may be embarrassed or reluctant to divulge their true concerns or feelings directly to the doctor. They may unintentionally send out signals through their body language, facial expressions or tone of voice which are incongruent with the content of what they are saying. The patient may even intentionally drop verbal cues in the hope that the listener enquires and explores them further.

Non-verbal cues

Doctors should aim to pickup on any non-verbal cues from the moment the patient enters into the room. Pay particular attention to gestures, movements and body language that the patient may exhibit.

A patient may use facial expressions, such as raising their eyebrows to express surprise or biting their lip when nervous, to signal that they are not in agreement with something you have said. A patient whose hand is clenched in a fist may be upset or angry whilst a patient making poor eye contact and fidgeting with their fingers may be anxious.

The manner in which a patient uses their tone of voice, pace of speech, and emphasis on words may dramatically alter the intended meaning. Take for example the word 'fine'. A patient who is genuinely feeling well when asked how they are would normally say *'I am fine'* in a confident and enthusiastic manner. On the other hand, someone who is feeling down and low will often reply *'I am fine'* in a low-pitched and lacklustre way. Although the two replies are verbally identical, the way in which they were expressed has a huge bearing on the intended meaning.

Verbal cues

Verbal cues are often subtly introduced by the patient for the doctor to recognise and pursue. They may add an extra dimension to the history and reveal additional patient concerns. If missed by the doctor, the patient is likely to reintroduce the cue, perhaps phrased in a different way, until it is acknowledged. Patients may be left disappointed if these cues are continually missed or ignored. Consider the following example:

Doctor:	'So, just to summarise what you've told me. You have had this niggling dry cough for the past six months. However, apart from that you have been quite well and not losing weight, and all the blood tests have been normal.'
Patient:	'Yeah, I know this cough's probably nothing . . . I mean like I'm only young and I've cut my smoking right down. It's probably nothing serious . . .'
Doctor:	'Well, you are quite correct. It's unlikely to be anything serious . . .'
Patient:	'Well, I have smoked since I was really young and I do live in house full of smokers. That could cause some damage couldn't it?'
Doctor:	'OK. You are obviously quite worried about the effects of smoking. Is there anything specific that may be troubling you?'
Patient:	'Well, my dad did die from lung cancer recently . . .'

Consultation framework

As no two doctors or patients are alike, one would assume that the doctor–patient consultation would be an unpredictable affair. In reality the consultation flows through a number of sequential stages that include introduction, information gathering, decision making, explaining, as well as closing up. This model is a simple yet effective approach in dealing with consultations.

This framework should not be considered as rigid; rather, the consultation should be permitted to flow through these phases at a natural pace that both parties are comfortable with.

Consultation setting

The environment in which you conduct your consultation with the patient can affect its direction and course. Attempts should be made to create an ideal atmosphere that is conducive for communication. Factors such as the general ambience of the room (temperature, lighting), level of privacy, presence of instrumentation and seating arrangement, should be optimised prior to commencing the consultation.

Ambience

Entering a room that is either too hot or too cold may make the patient feel uncomfortable even before the conversation has started. Coldness may make the patient feel unwelcomed, whereas a hot, stuffy atmosphere may choke the patient and unsettle them. A room that lacks natural light may exude negativity and feelings of gloominess. It is important, therefore, to take a few moments to adjust the heating and lighting in the room to create a warm and hospitable atmosphere.

Equipment and clutter

You should try to make your consultation room as clutter free as possible to reduce any distractions. Clutter, particularly on the desk, may be an unwanted distraction that may obscure the line-of-sight with the patient and interfere with maintaining good eye contact. Try to ensure that only essential equipment that is used day-to-day is present whilst non-essential items are stored away out of sight.

Seating arrangements

Classically, interviews are conducted across a desk. The desk, although convenient for organising documents and stationery, may create distance between yourself and the patient, thus impeding communication. It may also reinforce the stereotype of an authoritarian doctor, characteristic of a doctor-centred approach.

For this reason, the patient should be seated in a position that is not directly opposite the doctor. Instead, they should be seated across one corner of the desk. This will help both parties to be in closer proximity and encourage good eye contact and rapport.

Privacy

Patients sometimes attend their doctor with intimate and often highly embarrassing complaints. They expect that the information they divulge will be kept confidential and private, not open to others. Violation of this trust may have a terminal effect on the doctor–patient relationship. As a result, every attempt should be made to try to maintain the patient's privacy.

In an outpatient clinic or general practice setting, adequate privacy can usually be ensured by shutting the door or drawing the curtains. Privacy within an inpatient setting is usually harder to achieve unless the patient is situated in a side room. The absence of privacy within a ward cubicle, with only curtains acting as a non-soundproof barrier, is unlikely to fill the patient with enough confidence to impart information of a personal or sensitive nature. This may be compounded by the fact that wards are often noisy places and doctors on ward rounds may have to raise their voices to be heard. In so doing, patients in adjacent cubicles may inadvertently be privy to personal patient information. Hence, it may be an idea in such a setting to lower your voice and move closer to the patient to ensure that privacy is maintained.

Introducing yourself and establishing rapport

When seeing a patient for the first time, their initial impression of you may play an important role in shaping how the doctor–patient relationship develops. How you introduce yourself to the patient, greet and welcome them may leave a lasting impression in the patient's mind.

Rapport

Rapport is the ability to develop a common understanding with an individual that engenders mutual trust and respect. It often brings people closer together permitting the free exchange of honest ideas and emotions.

The process of establishing rapport should start with non-verbal actions such as early eye contact, smiling and handshaking. It should progress on to verbally introducing yourself as well as enquiring about the patient's general well-being.

Rapport should be maintained throughout the duration of the consultation and not be solely restricted to the early introductions. This can be achieved by showing a genuine interest in what the patient is saying, mirroring body language and matching the patient's pace and tone of speech.

Nodding, smiling and good eye contact work to encourage the patient's engagement and help build rapport.

Empathy

Empathy is the ability to share an individual's feelings and emotions whilst appreciating their point of view. Students often misunderstand the word empathy to simply mean feeling sorry for someone (i.e. being sympathetic). However, this understanding is far too simplistic.

Empathy implies feeling genuine compassion towards another person. It involves acknowledging their emotional state before making an empathic response befitting the situation. It is usually expressed verbally and reinforced with non-verbal communication. This may include facial expressions denoting concern and sorrow whilst offering a few comforting words. Often a simple action such as offering a box of tissues or a tender touch may encapsulate the moment better than any statements that you could make.

A person who is sympathetic but not truly empathic may come across as false and artificial. They may appear to be cold and insincere, dismantling any rapport that has already been built. Consider the example below of a sympathetic response:

Patient: 'I have been really upset since my stroke. I am now wheelchair bound and I can't visit my grandchildren . . .' (*Patient tearful*)

Doctor: 'That's sad to hear . . . How can I help you today?'

Contrast this with an empathic response:

Doctor: 'I am really sorry to hear that. It must be hard for you. (*Doctor offers tissues to the patient*) 'Is there anything that I can do to make things easier?'

Patient: 'Yes, it's been really hard. It's making me feel really down and depressed and has affected my sleep. That's why I have come to see you today.'

Introduction

Although it may seem obvious, it is important to have a good introductory statement. The opening phrase can go a long way in making the patient feel at ease and unrushed, and will contribute to the doctor–patient relationship. If you have not met the patient before, you should formally introduce yourself stating your name and grade of training before confirming the patient's details.

Doctor: 'Hello, I'm Dr Shaun Edwards. I am one of the medical doctors here. Are you Mr James?'

Patient:	'Yes, I am.'
Doctor:	'Pleased to meet you, do come in and take a seat.'

Information gathering

Patients attend their doctor for a variety of reasons. More often than not, they present with symptoms that they wish to have remedied. However, these symptoms usually do not occur in isolation. They are often entwined with complex psycho-social circumstances that directly impact upon the patient's quality of life. It is the doctor's job to make an attempt to unravel these issues and arrive at an accurate diagnosis.

Opening question

When you first begin the consultation, you should try to use questions that will encourage the patient to describe the problem in their own words. For most patients, visiting the doctor can be an anxiety-provoking experience. They may have already prepared a short speech of what they want to say and rehearsed this several times before they came to see you. Usually, a large proportion of the information that you require to make a diagnosis will be contained in this monologue.

By starting off the consultation with a series of narrow closed questions a patient will be forced into a sequence of 'yes' and 'no' answers, limited by your line of questioning. Using open questions such as *'What brought you here today?'* or *'How can I help you?'* will instead hand the initiative back to the patient and give them the opportunity to speak freely.

Allow the patient the freedom to talk uninterrupted until they come to a natural end. You may worry about what to do if the patient rambles on for 10 minutes. However, experience shows that patients on average only speak for around a minute and rarely exceed this. This is known as 'the golden minute'. Apart from being heard, the patient will appreciate the fact that they were actively listened to and given the chance to air their views without interruption.

Although you may feel tempted to interject whilst the patient is talking, apart from appearing rude, this may derail the patient's train of thought. Instead, it is better for you to make a mental note of any important questions and bring them up later for discussion.

Questioning

Open and closed questions are tools a doctor uses to find out more about the patient's presenting complaint. In isolation, neither approach is particularly helpful. However, when used together correctly they can be extremely productive.

Open questions

Open questions should primarily be used earlier on in the consultation. They allow the patient to express their story in their own words, as well as communicate their thoughts and emotions. Patients tend to give their accounts in a chronological order and in a manner that allows the listener to picture their experiences vividly and understand the context in which they occurred. The patient is also naturally inclined towards mentioning how each problem has affected their life and how it is a source of worry and concern to them. In many ways, the patient's story often negates the needs for a barrage of closed questions later on. Consider the following example of a doctor using closed questions from the outset of the consultation.

Doctor:	'What's been the problem?'
Patient:	'I feel a bit fuzzy in the head, Doctor.'
Doctor:	'Oh, you mean dizzy?'
Patient:	'Well, not really . . . yes perhaps . . .'
Doctor:	'So is the room spinning around you or do you just feel faint?'
Patient:	'Well, I'm not sure.'
Doctor:	'OK. Do you feel it when you stand up?'
Patient:	'Well, it is there when I stand up, but . . .'
Doctor:	'Good. It sounds as if you are suffering with postural hypotension. This is when your blood pressure falls as you stand up. You need to drink more in this hot weather as you are probably dehydrated as well. Does that make sense?'
Patient:	'Erm . . . yes . . . I think.'

Consider an alternative approach by using open questions early on in the consultation.

Doctor:	'So tell me, what seems to be the problem?'
Patient:	'I feel a bit fuzzy in the head, Doctor.'
Doctor:	'OK. Go on . . .'
Patient:	'Well, it started four days ago. I remember that day my hayfever was really bad. My brother's also got hay-fever so he suggested I take some anti-histamines. Anyway, since then I've found I can't really concentrate and I feel drowsy all the time. I'm a truck driver and usually I have no problem with long distances, but yesterday I found I was almost nodding off at the wheel!'
Doctor:	'I see. So how did you feel before taking the tablets?'
Patient:	'Well, apart from the hayfever, I was fine.'

Closed questions

Closed questions have a poor reputation because of their association with a doctor-centred approach. In the past they may have been used inappropriately by doctors to control and lead the consultation, limiting the opportunity for the patient to talk in order to expedite proceedings. However, if closed questions are used correctly they may add important detail and clarity to what the patient has said. They should be used nearer to the end of the consultation to home in on specific aspects of the story.

Leading questions

Leading questions are a form of closed questions that are phrased in such a way to seek out an intended response. They are biased towards a doctor-set agenda and limit the patient's ability to speak honestly. As they lead the patient into answering in a particular way, they contribute towards producing potentially inaccurate information. Below are examples of some leading questions and alternative ways of phrasing them.

Leading: 'You aren't a smoker, are you?'
Non-leading: 'Do you smoke?'
Leading: 'Have you stopped drinking excessively?'
Non-leading: 'How much alcohol do you drink at the moment?'
Leading: 'I really want to refer you to the surgeons, are you OK with that?'
Non-leading: 'How would you feel about being referred to the surgeons?'
Leading: 'You don't want me to give you another painkiller, do you?'
Non-leading: 'How do you feel about being prescribed more pain relief?'
Leading: 'Right, it's fair to assume there are no other problems today?'
Non-leading: 'Is there anything else that you wanted to talk about today?'

Complex questions

When questioning the patient, it is best to use simple and specific questions that leave no room for ambiguity. Employing unnecessarily complicated and long-winded questions are likely to confuse the patient and give you an unsatisfactory response.

Doctor: 'Do you find that previously, you may have enjoyed something like going to the pub for example, although I'm not saying that you do like the pub or drink alcohol, but that now you would rather not go? I mean this only by way of example and I don't mean that you binge drink or anything. Is that the case with you or not?'

Clearly, the doctor will confuse the patient with this style of questioning and may even inadvertently offend the patient. All of this could have been avoided by being precise and to the point.

Doctor: 'Do you find that you are no longer enjoying things that you previously did enjoy, such as going out to the pub?'

Another way in which questions may seem to be unnecessarily complicated is by posing a number of queries within a single question. This often occurs if the doctor has a sudden rush of ideas and hurries along with the questioning without pausing to think. Consider the following example:

Doctor: 'Did the pain come on suddenly or gradually or does anything make it better or worse?'

Any answer to the above question is likely to be meaningless as it has too many variables. Only one query should be posed to the patient at a time and a response should be sought before moving on to the next question.

Exploring the patient's presenting complaint

If the patient has attended with a medical complaint it is important to take a thorough medical history about each relevant symptom. This should include history of the complaint, past medical history, drug history, social history and family history. Do not forget to perform a general systems enquiry which will help uncover any allied symptoms.

Understanding the patient's perspective

Establishing the patient's perspective regarding their medical problem is an essential aspect of any consultation. Two patients may suffer from the same condition but experience its effects differently. Often the effect of the disease on the patient's quality of life is more concerning to them than the illness itself. By eliciting the patient's own ideas and concerns about their illness, the doctor is able to contextualise the problem as well as personalise the management plan accordingly. This also helps the patient feel that they are actively involved in the decision-making process and that their opinions are valued.

Be careful during the consultation, about hastily trying to establish the patient's perspective of their symptoms. Patients may freeze when directly asked for their thoughts before good rapport has been developed. Choose a time to raise these questions when it feels natural and appropriate to do so.

Ideas

Diseases can often be life-changing events, bringing anxiety and concern to the sufferer. Patients often try to make sense of and rationalise their problems to the best of their ability. This process may be influenced by the individual's own cultural background and norms, degree of medical knowledge or through the experiences of others. Hence, a patient may develop an inaccurate understanding about their condition which conflicts with current medical practice.

It is advisable to try to elicit these beliefs earlier on in the consultation. As these ideas may be held dear to the patient, you should be careful not to dismiss them outright, however far-fetched they may sound. Instead, you should initially acknowledge them before attempting to correct them later on in a sensitive manner. An appropriate time to undertake this may be during your explanatory phase of the consultation. You may find the following phrases useful when eliciting the patient's ideas:

'Tell me what you think is causing your problem?'
'Have you any idea as to why it happened?'
'Do you have an explanation or any theories about it?'

Concerns

It is easy to assume that a patient's main concern is simply to be given a diagnosis of their problem. More often than not, the anxieties held by the patient are not about simply reaching a diagnosis *per se* but rather about excluding serious pathology, such as cancer. Other concerns that rank highly in the patient's agenda include the impact of the illness upon the patient's life, as well as worries about premature death.

Failing to deal with these concerns may leave the patient feeling discontented and unhappy that the reason for their attendance had not been addressed. The phrases below are some examples of ways one can elicit a patient's concerns:

'Do you have any specific concerns about your symptoms?'
'Are you worried in any way about what you are experiencing?'
'Do you have any anxieties about it?'

Expectations

Based upon their ideas and concerns about their illness, a patient may have formed expectations about what the clinician should do for them. They may expect to be sent for more invasive tests and investigations, referred for specialist input, or be commenced on a specific treatment regime that they may have recently read about. Failure to elicit these expectations may lead to a disagreement between the patient and physician as to the best course of action.

Although a patient's expectations may clash with your professional judgement, it is important to take them on board before negotiating a shared management plan. In most cases, by explaining the disease process and treatment options available, the patient should develop a clearer picture of what their illness entails and revise their expectations accordingly. You may wish to determine the patient's expectations by asking:

> *'What did you think might be the next course of action?'*
> *'Did you come here with any expectations as to what should be done?'*
> *'How might I best help you with this problem?'*
> *'What were you hoping to happen next?'*

Examination

Depending on the presenting symptoms you should perform a focused physical examination of that particular system as relevant. This may reveal important signs that corroborate with the history you have elicited. If the patient presents with a psychological complaint, it may be prudent to complete a full psychiatric assessment including suicidal risk and self-harm.

Decision making

By now, you should have collected a wealth of information about the patient's reason for attendance and their presenting complaint. You should have also gained some useful insight into the patient's beliefs, worries and concerns. Collating this with your examination findings, you should be ready to formulate a working diagnosis with a list of possible differentials. Your task now is to communicate this to the patient effectively and explain to them what you believe should be the next course of action.

Explanation

Perhaps the most significant part of the consultation for the patient is the explanatory stage. The patient may have spent considerable effort explaining their problems, at times opening up intimate and embarrassing subjects, in the hope that you, the physician, would be able to diagnose and treat them.

Your medical training should have grounded you well in the ability to diagnose and treat patients. It is easy to assume that this is the only skill required to make a good doctor. However, in reality this is only part of the story. Without engaging the patient, any management plan that you formulate may not be accepted or implemented correctly.

You should make every effort to try to explain the diagnosis to the patient in a way that they can understand. Although this may sound simple enough, it often takes time and practice to perfect. By employing a few techniques, such as avoiding medical jargon, spacing out the information and checking understanding, you will become more confident and more competent in explaining complex medical conditions.

Organising the information

To aid the patient's understanding and avoid miscommunication, the information you give to the patient should be broken down into small digestible chunks. After each chunk, pause briefly to allow the patient time to process the information and reflect upon it. It may also be an idea to observe the patient's face for any cues that suggest they might not have completely understood what you have said.

In addition, your explanation should be devoid of any medical jargon or complex terminologies that may create confusion. It may be an idea to have thought out ways to phrase your explanation succinctly and rehearsed it before the consultation has even begun. Consider the following example of a doctor explaining asthma:

Doctor: 'Asthma is when the muscles in your bronchioles constrict due to an external allergen triggering an inflammatory process. This constriction reduces the diameter of your bronchioles thereby decreasing the ability for oxygen to flow and resulting in a high-pitched wheeze.'

The above explanation is replete with terms that are privy to the medical profession but largely unknown to the general public. Such an explanation would confuse rather than help the patient's understanding. An alternative approach could be:

Doctor: 'After considering what you told me and the flow test that you have just performed, I think you might be suffering from asthma.
PAUSE
'Asthma is a condition in which there is narrowing of the small airways in your lungs making it hard for air to flow through.
PAUSE
'It is thought that things called allergens may cause the muscles in your airway to tighten. When this happens you may notice that you are short of breath and may even cough.
PAUSE
'As air passes through these narrowed tubes it produces a sound that can be heard as a wheeze.'

Addressing cues and concerns

It is easy to forget, when motoring through your explanation, the real reason for the patient's attendance. As mentioned earlier, patients often attend with specific concerns that they wish to have addressed. By dealing with these concerns head on you will be able to tackle the patient's agenda and improve satisfaction in the consultation. Reinforce what you have said by incorporating the patient's ideas into your explanation and correct any misunderstandings they may hold. You may wish to ask:

> *'You mentioned previously that you were worried about . . .'*
> *'Going back to what you said earlier about your job . . .'*

During the explanatory phase of the consultation new cues may have cropped up. The patient may be confused as to what has been said, want clarification on a particular matter or may simply be overwhelmed with the amount of information given. If the patient appears anxious or worried, it may warrant further exploration. Offer the patient the chance to express themselves by asking:

> *'You looked a little unhappy when I was mentioning . . .'*
> *'I could tell that you seemed a little anxious about the diagnosis . . .'*

Check understanding

It may be all well and good to deliver a lengthy explanation to the patient believing that they have absorbed and retained everything that you have said. The reality is that patients often retain very little information when being lectured to. To assist information retention, it may be helpful to intersperse your explanation with short breaks to check the patient's understanding. The following phrases may be helpful in this regard:

> *'Are you happy with what I have said so far?'*
> *'Is that OK? Do you want me to go on?'*

Shared management plan

In the past, the doctor-centred approach involved the physician dictating a set of instructions to the patient to follow religiously. Superficially, the doctor may appear to be confident and knowledgeable in the eyes of the patient. Therefore, one would expect that the patient would be fully compliant with such diktats. However, research shows that this is not the case. Patients visit their doctor with an agenda that is shaped by a complex mix of health beliefs, concerns, worries and expectations. They expect their views will be heard, listened to, and acted upon. By ignoring this and imposing your own agenda, you are likely to antagonise them and cause a breakdown in communication.

A more balanced approach would be to regard your patient as a partner in the management plan. Inform them of the available treatment and management options, and give them time to appraise each one. Offer them information about individual pros and cons and possible adverse outcomes. Encourage the patient to actively contribute to the management plan by asking for their thoughts, ideas and preferences.

The patient should now be in a position to make an informed decision. Depending on how well you have explained yourself, the patient should be more open and agreeable to your advice. If however, despite your efforts the patient is still in disagreement with you, you should try to negotiate a compromise that is most acceptable to both parties.

Closing up

You are now approaching the end of the consultation. Before departing you should summarise back the key points to the patient, check their understanding of the information given, and agree on a date for a follow-up appointment.

Summarising back

By this time many issues will have been discussed in some detail and both parties' concentration may be waning. It is easy to presume that the patient has retained all that you have said. In reality, the patient is more than likely to be overwhelmed and suffering from information overload.

Summarising back to the patient will give you an opportunity to recap key points and check the patient's understanding. It will also act as a signpost to the patient that the consultation is drawing to a close.

The first part of your summary should include a brief synopsis of the information you have gathered from the patient. This should include the initial complaint, a brief history, the effects on their life and their ideas and concerns pertaining to it. Check with the patient that this information is accurate and offer them an opportunity to correct and amend if they see fit. If, in the rare event you realise that the information you have collected is grossly inaccurate, then you may need to revisit the history-taking phase of the consultation.

Doctor: 'Mrs Johnson, I would like to go over a few things that you have said to make sure that I have understood you clearly. Is that alright?'

Patient: 'Yes, no problem.'

Doctor: 'You mentioned that for the past six months you have been feeling more tired than usual and that your energy levels have diminished considerably. More recently, you have also noticed that your hands and elbows often feel stiff and more painful, worse in the morning and better in the evening. Is that right?'

19

Patient:	'Yes, that's correct.'
Doctor:	'Your mother and aunt both suffer from rheumatoid arthritis, and you are concerned that you may also now be affected.'
Patient:	'Yes, Doctor.'
Doctor:	'Is there anything that you wished to add?'
Patient:	'Only that it is really affecting my relationship with my husband.'
Doctor:	'Ah yes, of course! Thank you for reminding me.'

Having confirmed that the information you gathered is correct you should now proceed to summarise back the shared management plan.

Doctor:	'Based upon what you have told me, I believe that you may be suffering from arthritis. We have agreed to carry out a few blood tests to confirm what type of arthritis this may be. Depending on these results you may need to see a specialist. Are you happy with that?'

Encourage questions

Before you close, ask the patient if there is anything they would like to mention. Ideally, you would have already addressed most of the patient's immediate questions in your explanation. However, it is good practice to do a final check that the patient does not hold any unattended concerns or have anything else to add.

Thank the patient and close the consultation

One of the best ways to signal that the consultation has come to an end is to thank the patient and give a parting statement. It may, if appropriate, be accompanied by a non-verbal cue such as standing up or offering your hand by way of a handshake. Be careful, however, not to overtone your gestures in a way that could be interpreted as being rude and discourteous, making the patient feel unwelcomed and ushered to the door. Suitable closing up phrases include:

Doctor:	'Well thank you, Mr Edwards for coming today. I hope that these tablets do the trick and I look forward to seeing you again in the future.'
Doctor:	'Thank you, Mrs Jones. I hope things turn out for the best. I will be in touch soon.'
Doctor:	'OK then, Mr Smith. Thank you for coming. Let us know if you have any more problems.'

CHAPTER 2

Breaking bad news

All doctors will at some point in their careers have to break bad news to patients or their relatives. It may well be that you are required to inform a family member of an unexpected death or explain a diagnosis of cancer to a young patient. Someone must ultimately take the responsibility to impart this information and more often than not it will be you, the junior doctor.

Breaking bad news compassionately is the art of conveying information that people do not wish to hear. Doctors who have received inadequate instruction in this skill during the course of their medical training may feel anxious and worried about undertaking this task and deflect the responsibility to a more senior colleague.

They may be reluctant to put themselves forward because of a fear of being blamed and a worry that they will give inaccurate information. They may be concerned about how the patient might react, or be anxious about being too emotionally embroiled. By having limited exposure to these situations, they will not gain the opportunity to refine and improve their expertise in this skill.

Performing this skill well involves being able to give clear and unambiguous advice whilst remaining sensitive, tactful and honest. It is a skill which improves with experience and above all, practice. Adhering to some fundamental principles will usually make this task easier and provide a structure with which you can approach different scenarios.

Hopefully, through the course of this chapter, you will begin to appreciate that breaking bad news is an art that can be learnt. If used correctly you will be able to instil trust and confidence in your patient, prepare them for what may lie ahead, and avert potential litigious proceedings from being brought against you.

The consultation: breaking bad news

Before breaking bad news, you should formulate a clear plan in your mind as to how you will approach this, to help ensure that you do not miss anything important in the consultation or give out any contradictory messages. The exact approach is not critical and a certain degree of flexibility is often needed with varying scenarios.

Different patients respond in different ways when receiving bad news. Some may react with alarm and despair, breaking into a flood of tears, whilst others may fall into an apparent trance or drown in a sea of silence. Hence, it is important to remain flexible in your approach and tailor the consultation depending on your knowledge about the patient and their condition.

Preparation

Irrespective of the situation you find yourself in, whether real life or under exam conditions, always start by gaining as much information as possible about the patient's problem.

If you are in a clinic, the correspondence section of the notes is a good way of swiftly reviewing the history, investigations and treatments the patient has had to date. In an examination situation, be sure to carefully read and digest the clinical vignette before entering the station. You are unlikely to impress the examiner by interrupting the flow of the consultation either by repeatedly checking the clinical details or by spending undue time reviewing the presenting complaint with the actor.

After you have gathered sufficient information, spend a few moments collecting your thoughts and emotions before starting. Try to hypothesise a list of possible questions that you may be asked and prepare responses for these. Be prepared to be frank and open in saying, *'I don't know'* to a question that you feel is beyond your level of expertise. More often than not, poor delivery of bad news is simply due to a lack of preparation.

Setting the scene

The setting in which you the break bad news is also extremely important. Despite time constraints, you should make an effort to locate an appropriate setting that would assist the process. Most wards have day rooms which can help to create a calm and private environment. However, when they are not available, you may have to break bad news at the bedside. In such a situation, simple but effective measures such as closing curtains, ensuring adequate seating and removing obvious distractions (such as bed pans and open sputum pots), help to maintain the patient's privacy and dignity. In addition, consider handing your bleep to a colleague to avoid any unnecessary interruptions whilst you are with the patient.

Involving friends and relatives

In real life, it may be advisable for the patient to be accompanied by a close relative when receiving the bad news. If the patient attends the consultation alone, check that they have not left someone waiting outside for them. In most cases, with the patient's consent, it is easier for them to deal with the bad news if a close relative is at hand. Asking the patient if they would like to bring a relative to the consultation is also a useful cue that you will be imparting some important information.

It may be the case that the patient is too unwell to comprehend what is being discussed and you have to break the news to a family member instead. In such situations it is important to ascertain who that person is and how they are related to the patient. By not doing so, you may impart sensitive information to a casual friend and inadvertently break the patient's right to confidentiality.

Introducing yourself and establishing rapport

It is important to introduce yourself clearly to the patient or relative, stating your name and position. You should do this even if you have had previous encounters with the patient and believe that they already know who you are. This will help maintain the formality of the occasion. An informal introduction may be misinterpreted as a cue that good news rather than bad is to be received.

Having introduced yourself to the patient, you should try to develop a good rapport with them. This will engender trust and confidence in you and the advice you will give. An example of this would be to ask open-ended questions to the patient such as: *'How have you been today?'* or *'How was your journey to the hospital?'*

When listening to the patient's response, try to demonstrate to them that you have an active interest in what they are saying. Observe the patient for any non-verbal cues that could reflect their current state of mind. Are they apprehensive or fearful? Do they appear calm and collected? You may have to tailor the consultation according to how the patient is feeling.

Understanding the patient's perspective

You should make some effort to establish the patient's awareness and understanding about their condition prior to breaking the bad news. This will help you appreciate how much the patient already knows and give you an insight into any concerns they may have.

Ideas: what is the patient's current understanding of events?

You must never walk into a consultation with preconceptions about the patient, especially when preparing to break bad news. A helpful way of gauging how you should go about breaking bad news would be to first establish what the patient already knows. Often the patient knows little else except that they are waiting for the results of some recent blood tests. They may be innocently oblivious to the magnitude of the news that you are about to give.

Check the patient's level of understanding about their condition by asking open questions such as:

'Do you have any ideas about what may be causing your symptoms?'
'Have you had any thoughts about what is going on?'

Concerns: is the patient worried about anything in particular?

Eliciting the patient's concerns is of vital importance to the doctor–patient relationship. It demonstrates a sympathetic and empathic approach and makes the patient feel that they are being listened to.

Do not automatically assume that the patient's sole worry is about what their diagnosis is. In many cases, patients may have already prepared themselves for the worst and are more concerned about practical issues such as inheritance or the care of a surviving spouse. Therefore, you should avoid using closed questions when eliciting their concerns. Instead, use open questions to allow the patient to speak freely and tell you what is really troubling them. Useful phrases that may help you include:

'Is there anything in particular that is worrying you?'
'Do you have any particular concerns you would like to raise with me today?'

Breaking the bad news

Having established the patient's own ideas and concerns about their illness, it may now be an appropriate time to prepare the patient to receive the bad news. Breaking bad news should be performed in stages to ease the patient through this challenging process. By forewarning the patient, you will alert them that some difficult news is forthcoming.

Signposts and warning shots

Breaking bad news suddenly can generate an unexpected response from the patient. It may stun them into a stupor, numbing their senses from absorbing any further information. For this reason, it is advisable to fire 'warning shots' to the patient to indicate that some unpleasant news is about to follow.

Unwittingly, you may have already prepared the ground work for this. For example, by taking the patient to a separate room, sitting them down and offering them a cup of coffee, this may have heightened their awareness that something significant is about to be discussed. However, do not take this for granted as the patient may interpret such behaviour as simple courtesy and professionalism. Hence, it may be helpful to verbally reinforce the warning shots by saying something such as:

'I'm afraid I have some difficult news to tell you . . .'
'I'm sorry to say that the results are more serious than we had hoped . . .'

This acts as a prelude to the bad news and affords the patient some time to prepare themselves for what you are about to tell them. It also allows them to open up, engage and be less defensive when receiving the news. Imagine the reaction you would get if you were to hastily break the bad news and say bluntly:

Doctor:	'So you've come today to find out your blood results. Well . . . the results show you have cancer! What should we do about it?'
Patient:	'What?! I thought I was here to pick up my prescription.'

After you have signalled to the patient that bad news is about to follow, pause and allow them to respond. They may tell you their worst fears or pre-empt what you are about to say. They may even burst into tears. Whatever the case, give the patient time and wait for a cue that suggests that they are ready to carry on.

Imparting the news

There is no easy way to break bad news to the patient. However, there are techniques and approaches to help you impart the information in a sensitive, caring and empathic way. In so doing, you are likely to influence the response of the patient in a positive way and less likely to induce a negative knee-jerk reaction.

Body language

It is important to check your own positioning and posture, if you already have not done so. An open posture conveys warmth, trust and receptiveness and encourages the patient to engage with you. Simple things such as sitting closer to the patient and at the same level may help establish a stronger bond between you and the patient.

Pauses

When delivering the bad news, it is tempting to rush through, in the hope that you will get it over and done with quickly. Doctors often think that by getting the news out in the open they have performed their duty and absolved their responsibility to the patient. Invariably, this will cause more harm than good. Instead, you should pace the delivery of information to the patient by breaking it into short chunks. Allow for regular pauses that will give the patient time to digest and react to what has been said. Consider the example below:

Doctor:	'I'm afraid the scan results are not what we hoped for.'
	PAUSE
Patient:	'In what way?'
Doctor:	'They show that the initial problem has spread.'
	PAUSE
Patient:	'You mean the cancer has spread?'
Doctor:	'Yes, I'm afraid it has.'
	PAUSE
Patient:	'So will that explain the headaches I've been having?'
Doctor:	'I believe so, yes.'
	PAUSE
Patient:	'Oh my God. Has it spread to my brain?'
Doctor:	'Yes, I'm afraid it has.'

In a pressured clinic or examination situation, it may be tempting for you to cut corners and break the news all at once, saying:

Doctor: 'I'm afraid the scan results show that your lung cancer has spread to the brain and caused several nasty new cancerous growths. This is the cause of your headaches. I am sorry.'

As you can imagine, such an abrupt and insensitive approach will not only worsen the discomfort and distress of the patient but would also open up a Pandora's box of emotions.

Avoiding medical jargon

When you are communicating with patients, it is important to use language and terms that the patient will understand and be familiar with. This will help prevent confusion or any embarrassing miscommunications.

For example, if you were to tell a patient that they had a mesothelioma, they may feel falsely reassured that they do not have lung cancer. Whilst your information is clinically correct, the patient may not fully understand the diagnosis. Consider how you would manage the following situation:

Doctor:	'We got the results of your scan and it shows a breast carcinoma.'
	PAUSE
Patient:	'Oh, that's a relief. I haven't got breast cancer then!'
Doctor:	'Well . . .?'

Patient's response to the bad news

Having broken the bad news, you may think that the tricky part is over and that you can now relax. Unfortunately, this is not the case as the patient's response to the news may at times be paralysing.

The patient's reaction is likely to be an expression of grief, taking the form of crying, staring into space, or shouting angrily. The patient may even begin to blame you for what has happened or completely deny that they are unwell. Whatever the situation, allow the patient sufficient time to react and vent their frustration.

It is important that you maintain your professionalism even during these sensitive times and do not trivialise the patient's emotional response. Avoid being condescending towards the patient by saying such phrases as *'pull yourself together'*, or *'it will be OK'*. Rather, be compassionate to their plight whilst sensitively acknowledging their emotional state.

Crying

A common response following the receipt of bad news is for the patient to burst into tears and cry. This may vary in intensity from patient to patient. Some may wail out loudly, whilst others sob away quietly. If this happens, do not become unnerved and detach yourself from the patient. Rather, be empathic and acknowledge the patient's right to express their emotions. It may be appropriate to offer a box of tissues or a glass of water to help calm the patient down.

Anger

Another typical response you may face is for the patient is to become angry. Again this may vary in degree from patient to patient and from situation to situation. Patients may direct their anger at themselves or at you. It is always important to acknowledge their anger and attempt to defuse the situation in a calm and collected way. You may wish to say:

Doctor: 'You seem quite upset at the moment. That's perfectly understandable. However, I want you to know that I'm here to help.'

In the unlikely event that the patient becomes aggressive or threatening, the safest approach would be to tell the patient that you are feeling uncomfortable and that you may terminate the consultation. In most cases, this will be sufficient to defuse the intensity of the situation and make the patient realise the error of their ways.

Doctor: 'I understand that you are angry about what has happened.

	However, I am beginning to feel uneasy with your current behaviour towards me.'
	PATIENT STANDS UP AGGRESSIVELY SHOUTING
Doctor:	'I am now feeling more uncomfortable with how things are proceeding. I have to warn you that if you do not stop this behaviour I will have to end this meeting and leave the room.'

Silence

Some patients respond to bad news with a deafening silence. This can often be the most difficult of emotions to deal with. A patient sitting silently staring into space can unsettle even the most experienced of physicians. A possible way of resolving this dilemma is to ask the patient if they are OK to continue. You could say for example:

Doctor:	'I know this was totally unexpected . . . do you want me to carry on?'

Hopefully this will trigger some response from the patient allowing you to re-engage them in the consultation.

Giving more information

Once the patient has reacted to and accepted the news, they will probably want to know more information about their treatment options and prognosis. More often than not they will ask: *How long do I have to live, Doc?'* At this stage, you may not have access to specific information that will help you answer such questions. Also, you may not feel confident enough, due to lack of experience or expertise, to hazard a guess about the patient's future prospects. If you believe that this is outside your level of expertise you should never give false reassurances to the patient. Instead, be honest in your answer and offer to refer them to colleagues who are better versed in the relevant specialty. For example, you may wish to employ the following technique:

Patient:	'Is this the end, Doctor?'
Doctor:	'That is a very difficult question for me to answer and I don't want to give you any incorrect information. It may be best if I refer you to a colleague who is more specialised than me in this matter. They will be better equipped to answer any specific questions you have. Would you be happy with this?'
Patient:	'Yes. If you think so . . .'

In some unfortunate cases you may be required to explain to the patient that their condition is incurable. In such circumstances, you should use the same framework as described above, not forgetting to give small chunks of information and 'signpost' bad news as appropriate.

Patient: 'So I guess you'll be talking to the brain surgeons to get rid of these new growths?'

Doctor: 'I'm afraid surgery won't solve the problem.'
PAUSE

Patient: 'So you're telling me you aren't going to do anything?'

Doctor: 'Unfortunately, it is more serious than we had hoped. It looks as if surgery would not be able to cure you. However, I would like you to see one of the oncologists, who are the cancer specialists. They will be able to provide you with alternative options.'

Patient: 'If they won't operate, what's the point? What will they offer me?'

Doctor: 'They will aim to offer you either radiation treatment (radiotherapy) or medicines (chemotherapy) to try to shrink the cancer down. That should help with the headaches and vomiting you've been experiencing.'
PAUSE

Patient: 'More chemotherapy?'

Doctor: 'I'm afraid so. It appears that may be the case.'

Patient: 'Well as long as it gets rid of these cancers in my brain.'
PAUSE

Doctor: 'I'm sorry. It will only shrink the cancers. Unfortunately, they are unlikely to completely go away.'

Patient: 'So you can't cure them?'
PAUSE

Doctor: 'I'm afraid not. I'm really sorry.'

Of course, not all scenarios of breaking bad news involve incurable metastatic cancer. In many cases, there is realistic hope of success in treatment and good prospect of an unaltered quality of life. In these situations, you should reassure the patient and encourage them to be hopeful.

Doctor: 'I can see that you are quite upset at the moment as you have just found out you are diabetic. However, I would like to point out that diabetes is an illness which we can treat extremely effectively. As long as your blood sugar is well monitored and controlled, there is no reason why you can't continue to enjoy life normally.'

Eliciting further concerns

By now you will have broken the bad news and given the patient further information about what may happen next. It may be tempting to conclude the consultation on the assumption that the patient is content with what has been discussed. However, it is likely that the patient has developed new concerns as a result of the bad news. It is essential that you try to address these new concerns before allowing the patient to leave the consultation. If left unaddressed, such worries and anxieties may often simmer away and preoccupy the patient's thoughts.

Doctor: 'Now that you know that you have diabetes, is there anything in particular you are worried about?'

Patient: 'I am really worried about going blind . . .'

Doctor: 'Go on. Please tell me more . . .'

Discussing concerns at this stage will also allow the patient to reflect upon possible difficulties that may arise in the short, medium and long term. They may have to make important decisions, for example, about their living arrangements or finances, which may adversely affect their life. Prompting the patient to acknowledge these issues now will help them think about ways to address them in the future.

Establishing support strategies

It is more than likely that the primary concern of the patient would be how they will cope with the burdensome news that they have just received. The overwhelming shock of the bad news may leave the patient feeling desolate and lonely, with all their troubles and concerns on their shoulders. However, they often have good social networks or support from family, who can help them at this time of distress.

Try to ascertain from the patient whether they live alone or with family, and whether they have a close confidant with whom they can share their worries. Spend some time exploring this area as the patient may not wish to engage other people for fear of being an inconvenience. Reassure them that they do not have to suffer in silence and that friends and family are normally more than happy to help out in such times of need.

If the patient is truly alone, you may wish to consider contacting local services that are available to help. These may include counselling services, bereavement or patient support groups which have valuable experience in dealing with such problems.

Doctor: 'You have had a lot to take in today. Can I ask if you have anyone close who can help you through this difficult time?'

Patient: 'There is my wife but she is very sick. I do not want to burden her with this.'

Doctor: 'I am sorry to hear that your wife is sick. Would you prefer talking to someone else, like a counsellor? Do you think that may useful?'

Summarising back

A lot of information would have been given to the patient in a very short space of time. They are likely to be feeling quite emotional and struggling to keep up with what has been said. It is important therefore, that you check whether the patient has understood and retained the pertinent points of the consultation so that you can safely move on to discuss management plans.

Summarise the key points of the discussion and reflect them back to the patient. Specifically ask whether the information you have summed up is a fair representation of what has been said and whether the patient would like any further clarification.

Doctor: 'A lot has been mentioned today, and I'm sure you are feeling overwhelmed. I would like to just check that you have understood everything by summarising a few points. Would that be OK?'

Agreeing on a shared management plan

There is evidence to show that when a patient is engaged and involved in the decision-making process they are more likely to show concordance with the agreed management plan. This is particularly true when breaking bad news. The patient is the key participant in the process and their opinion must be sought and valued. Imagine a scenario where you have just broken news to a patient that they require radical surgery for a previously unknown bladder cancer and that the operation has been booked for next week. How would you expect the patient to respond if they were not consulted about it?

A better approach would be to inform the patient of the possible management options and seek their opinion on each. For example, a patient with end-stage liver cancer should be offered the choice as to whether they wish to spend their remaining time at home, in hospital or at a hospice. Be sure to tell the patient about the pros and cons of each option and give them time to arrive at a decision.

Follow-up and referring on

You may have mentioned that you will be referring the patient to a specialist to discuss further treatment and prognosis of their illness. However, it may be courteous to offer them an opportunity to see you again in a few weeks' time in order to discuss how they are coping, and suggest that, if they have not already done so, they ask a family member or friend to accompany them for emotional assistance and moral support.

Use the opportunity to remind the patient of other services available to them such as a counsellor, specialist nurse or their own GP who may be able to offer useful help and advice. By mentioning this towards the end of the consultation it may also act as cue that the consultation is drawing to a close.

Doctor:	'Our MacMillan nurses provide care and support for people with cancer. We can arrange for you to have a chat today or, if you would prefer, in a day or two once you have had a chance to think about things.'
Patient:	'Thank you, Doctor. Having thought about it, I might need someone else to talk to. I'm worried I can't cope.'
Doctor:	'I will get in touch with the MacMillan nurse for you. If there are any issues which you are struggling to deal with, we can also provide you with details of our counsellors. It is usually possible to arrange to see them at short notice.'
Patient:	'Yes, I'd like that too, thank you.'

Ending the consultation

You may find it hard to end the consultation having broken such difficult news. You may even feel partly responsible for the patient's emotional state. However, the patient needs time to digest and consider what you have told them. They may need a 'time out' to consolidate the information.

Try to allow the consultation to run its natural course and do not end it prematurely as this may make the patient feel that they are being forced out of the door and undo all your hard work in establishing rapport.

Housekeeping

Breaking bad news is one of the most emotionally draining and involving tasks that you will have to perform. Having just catered for all of the patient's wants and concerns, which may well have been quite challenging, you should not forget to take a brief time out to collect your own thoughts and emotions. Do not hesitate to approach friends or colleagues, if need be, to discuss your feelings. This may be a useful way of winding down and allowing you to address any lingering concerns that you may have.

Doctors are notoriously bad at looking after their own health needs and this may have a knock-on effect, not only on yourself, in terms of stress and becoming overworked, but also on your care for the patients that will follow.

FIRST CLINICAL SCENARIO

Breaking bad news to a patient

You will be required to break bad news to patients throughout your career. This may be in the context of an outpatient clinic, a GP surgery or even during an acute admission. Whatever the setting is the principles of breaking bad news remain the same. Try to fire a 'warning shot' before actually breaking the bad news. Allow the patient time to digest the information and give them ample space to express their emotions.

DOCTOR'S BRIEF

You are the Speciality Trainee in Emergency Medicine. You have been asked to speak to Mr Gould, a 78-year-old man who has been brought in by ambulance after being knocked over by a vehicle whilst crossing the road. Following a series of X-rays and CT scans, he is found to have a crush injury of his right leg and now requires a below-knee amputation. Mr Gould is otherwise very fit and well and is quite active for his age. Break the news to him that he will require an amputation.

ACTOR'S BRIEF *(if you are the doctor, please do not read)*

You are William Gould, a 78-year-old retired head teacher. Unfortunately, you were knocked over by a car earlier this evening. Apart from severe pain in your right leg, which you are unable to move, you do not recall any other problems. You suspect that your right leg is likely to be broken but are glad that you 'got off lightly' as you are not aware of anything else seriously wrong with you.

Although you have undergone several scans, you have not yet been informed what the results are. You expect to be in plaster for a number of months but think that the recovery process should be quite swift.

You lost your wife four years ago, and took up some new hobbies to keep you occupied, such as an outdoor walking group. However, you have booked tickets for an ocean cruise in nine months on the same date as your wedding anniversary. You have a fighting spirit and will respond to any challenge. What you are really dreading is being told that your recovery will take longer than expected and that you will miss your cruise.

If the doctor rushes through breaking the bad news, you will disengage and will not disclose personal information about your wife or hobbies.

SCENARIO WALK-THROUGH

INTRODUCE YOURSELF TO THE PATIENT	*Doctor:*	'Hello, Mr Gould. My name is Dr Joseph. I am one of the A&E doctors who has been involved in your care.'
	Mr Gould:	*'Hello, Doctor.'*
MAINTAIN PRIVACY WHILST BREAKING BAD NEWS	*Doctor:*	'I am pleased to meet you. Please excuse me for a few minutes as I need to hand over my bleep to a colleague.'
	Mr Gould:	*'OK, Doctor.'*

YOU SHUT THE CUBICLE CURTAINS AND HAND OVER YOUR BLEEP

OPEN QUESTION AND ESTABLISHING RAPPORT	*Doctor:*	'I'm very sorry to hear about what happened to you this evening. How are you feeling at the moment?'
	Mr Gould:	*'Well, to be honest, I feel a lot better than I should, I guess. I've had a very lucky escape. I suppose I should be grateful I only have a broken leg! That is assuming my leg is broken.'*
ESTABLISH PATIENT'S IDEAS	*Doctor:*	'Well, that is correct, you have fractured the bones of your lower leg. Do you know anything more about your injuries?'
	Mr Gould:	*'Oh, so that confirms it then. Well, I suppose I want to know how bad the fracture is and how long it will take to heal. There's a cruise I've booked at the end of the year and I don't want to miss it.'*
WARNING SHOT	*Doctor:*	'Mr Gould, unfortunately the injuries you have sustained appear to be more serious than we had expected . . .'
USE OF PAUSES	PAUSE	
	Mr Gould:	*'What do you mean?'*
BREAK THE NEWS IN STEPS	*Doctor:*	'I'm afraid that the accident has badly affected your right leg . . .'
	PAUSE	
	Mr Gould:	*'I don't understand, Doctor. It's going to be alright, isn't it?'*
	Doctor:	'The scan shows that the structures in your lower leg have been badly damaged and a simple operation will not help.'
	Mr Gould:	*'What! You are not operating then?'*

Doctor:	'Unfortunately, it appears that the injury is very severe and requires a below-knee amputation.
PAUSE	
	'I'm sorry, Mr Gould.'
Mr Gould:	'OH MY GOD. I can't believe it! There must be something you can do!'
PAUSE	
Doctor:	'I really am very sorry, Mr Gould . . .'

Patient sobs loudly . . . (Doctor offers a box of tissues and allows patient time to fully respond to the bad news)

<table>
<tr><td>ACKNOWLEDGES PATIENT'S EMOTIONAL STATE</td><td></td></tr>
</table>

Mr Gould:	'I don't know how I am going to cope. My outdoor pursuits, my travelling . . . its all that I have left since my wife died!'
Doctor:	'I realise this must come as a shock to you.'

EMPATHIC RESPONSE

DEMONSTRATE ACTIVE LISTENING

Mr Gould:	'Oh my God. The cruise . . . that was to remind me of our wedding anniversary. How will I go in this state? Its impossible!' (Patient cries)
Doctor:	'I can see that your wife meant a great deal to you and going on this cruise is very important. I can assure you that we will do everything we can to get you back to as near normal functioning as possible.'
Mr Gould:	'How? I won't be able to walk again once you remove my leg.'

GIVING SUPPORTIVE ADVICE

Doctor:	'Thankfully, you are in very good hands. People who have had leg amputations are now able to live near normal lives with a limb prosthesis. We have some very skilled physiotherapists who will work closely with you to improve your mobility.'
Mr Gould:	'That can't be the case. You're just saying that to lessen the blow.'
Doctor:	'No . . . really. I have personally been involved with a number of patients who have returned to their hobbies after being in a similar situation as yourself.'
Mr Gould:	'Well, if that's the case I won't take this lying down! If there is any chance of me getting on that cruise, I'll take it.'

CHECK FOR SUPPORT NETWORK	*Doctor:*	'Brilliant, I am really pleased to hear that. I must admit it is going to take a lot of hard work to get through this but I can see that you are quite determined. Can I ask if you have anyone close to you who can help you through this difficult time?'
	Mr Gould:	*'Yeah, there is my son who I am very close to. He can help me out with my day-to-day chores.'*
	Doctor:	'It's good to hear that you have someone to help you. That will be useful on your road to recovery.'
	Mr Gould:	*'Yes, he's very good to me.'*
SUMMARISE BACK	*Doctor:*	'Well . . . you have had a lot to take in today – do you mind if I go over a few things that we have discussed?'
	Mr Gould:	*'No, that's fine. It has been a very busy day indeed!'*
	Doctor:	'You were admitted to hospital following a road traffic accident. Unfortunately, you damaged your right leg quite badly and we are unable to save it.

PAUSE

'However despite this, we will try to provide you with a prosthetic limb and will work hard with you to get you back as close as possible to your normal function.'

Mr Gould: *'Yes, that seems to be the gist of it. Can I have some time alone please?'*

Doctor: 'Yes, of course. If you do have any questions or worries or simply want someone to talk to, just ask one of the nurses to bleep me.'

Mr Gould: *'Thanks, that's awfully kind.'*

Doctor: 'No problem. Take care.'

CONSULTATION END

SECOND CLINICAL SCENARIO

Breaking bad news to a relative

There are many occasions where you will be required to break bad news to relatives or carers for reasons other than the death of the patient. These may include a patient unconscious in ITU or a child diagnosed with a chronic illness such as leukaemia. The same structure for breaking bad news should be used when confronted with such a scenario.

DOCTOR'S BRIEF

You are the Foundation Year House Officer in Elderly Care. Mrs Dawson is an 82-year-old woman with dementia who was recently admitted onto your ward with chronic constipation and a recent episode of PR bleed. On routine examination, a hard abdominal mass was found and a CT scan confirmed metastatic malignancy. Her daughter, who is her main carer, has come in to find out about her mother's progress and has requested to speak to you. Inform the patient's daughter of the diagnosis.

ACTOR'S BRIEF *(if you are the doctor, please do not read)*

You are Sheila Davis, a 55-year-old woman who has been living with her mother for the last 20 years.

You are aware that your mother has had constipation for several months. Deep down you have been worried that there may be a possibility of cancer. However, you have tried to convince yourself that this is nothing sinister because the thought of losing your only family member is too much to handle. You are also worried that if your mother becomes poorly, you will not be able to cope with looking after her and keeping your stressful job.

Your life has been full of difficulties. Five years ago, your husband died tragically in a road accident. Six months ago you were diagnosed with type 2 diabetes and hypertension, which has been fairly well controlled. Your mother is the only family member you have. She is very close to you and has always been very supportive of you during your times of hardship.

You are an extremely private person and have discussed your personal circumstances with only a few of your closest friends. *You will not volunteer information about your past unless prompted to do so.*

SCENARIO WALK-THROUGH

INTRODUCE YOURSELF TO THE PATIENT'S RELATIVE	*Doctor:*	'Hello. My name is Dr Smith and I am one of the doctors looking after your mother, Mrs Dawson. Can I just confirm that you are Mrs Dawson's daughter?'
	Daughter:	'Yes, I'm Sheila Davis. Is everything alright with my mum?'
MAINTAIN PRIVACY WHILST BREAKING BAD NEWS	*Doctor:*	'I am pleased to meet you. The ward is very busy and noisy; would you prefer to go somewhere more private?'
	Daughter:	'Yes. That would be good.'

YOU TAKE THE DAUGHTER INTO THE DAY ROOM

OPEN QUESTION AND ESTABLISHING RAPPORT	*Doctor:*	'Your mother has been in hospital for the last few days. How do you think she is coping?'
	Daughter:	'I think she is doing alright, but I hoped that she would have returned home by now. Is anything the matter?'
ESTABLISH RELATIVE'S IDEAS	*Doctor:*	'She has been suffering with constipation for a while. Do you have any ideas as to what may be causing her symptoms?'
	Daughter:	'Well, mum has had constipation for the last few years and it's been getting worse and worse which has worried me. She has been in and out of the GP's surgery. I thought it may be because she hasn't been eating or moving around a lot recently.'
ESTABLISH RELATIVE'S CONCERNS	*Doctor:*	'Is there anything in particular that is worrying you about your mother's condition?'
DEMONSTRATE ACTIVE LISTENING, (EYE CONTACT, OPEN BODY POSTURE)	*Daughter:*	'I am worried that she is not her normal self any more. She doesn't talk as much and is tired all the time. I just don't know how to cope with her any more.'
SHOW EMPATHY AND ESTABLISH RELATIVE'S EXPECTATIONS	*Doctor:*	'I can see how this is very difficult for you. Maybe we can discuss ways of helping you? Was there anything else that you wanted to discuss with me today?'
	Daughter:	'Yes. I understand that mum had a scan yesterday. Do you know what it showed?'
	Doctor:	'Yes, your mum did have the scan yesterday and we have the preliminary reports.'

USE OF PAUSES	**PAUSE**

Doctor: 'Unfortunately, it is more serious than we had hoped . . .'

WARNING SHOT

PAUSE

Daughter: *'How Doctor?'*

Doctor: 'I am sorry to have to tell you that the CT scan has shown that the constipation that your mother has been suffering from is due to a growth in her bowel.'

BREAK THE NEWS USING SIMPLE, JARGON-FREE LANGUAGE

PAUSE

Daughter: *'Growth! You mean cancer, right?!'*

Doctor: 'Yes, unfortunately.'

(Daughter breaks down into tears)

SHOW EMPATHY AND MANAGE RELATIVE'S EMOTIONAL RESPONSE

Doctor: 'I am sorry I had to tell you this . . . Please, take some tissues and take as long as you need.'

Daughter: *'OH MY GOD . . . How did this happen? How am I going to cope? What am I going to do? I have got enough on my plate already.'*

PAUSE

Doctor: 'I know that this is a lot to take in. Is there anything I can help you with?'

DEMONSTRATE ACTIVE LISTENING

Daughter: *'My husband died a few years ago and I have recently been diagnosed with blood pressure and diabetes. And now I have been told my mum has cancer! How am I going to cope?'*

ACKNOWLEDGE RELATIVE'S ANXIETIES AND OFFER SUPPORT STRATEGIES

Doctor: 'I am sorry that all of these things have happened to you in recent times. I can see that you have been managing a lot of stress on your own. Maybe there are ways we can help you. There are a number of services available which can assist you in looking after your mother at home if you so wish?'

Daughter: *'I need more time to think about this. There is so much to take in.'*

CHECK FOR SUPPORT NETWORK

Doctor: 'I agree. This has been a difficult day for you. Is there anyone at home that you can speak to?'

Daughter: *'Yes. I have a very close friend whom I speak to about everything. I'll ring her when I get home.'*

	Doctor:	'We have a trained counsellor who is very good at giving constructive advice in these situations. Would you like to see her?'
	Daughter:	*'I think that is a good idea. However, I feel I need some time to think everything through first.'*
CHECK RELATIVE'S UNDERSTANDING OF INFORMATION GIVEN	Doctor:	'I think that would be ideal. A lot has been mentioned today, and I'm sure you feel overwhelmed by it all. Is it OK if I just go over some of the points we have discussed today?'
	Daughter:	*'Yes . . . please.'*
SUMMARISE BACK	Doctor:	'I am sorry to have had to inform you today that your mother was diagnosed with bowel cancer. I understand that you have had a difficult time recently. I will be speaking to a counsellor to get in touch with you. Is that OK?'
	Daughter	*'Yes.'*
OFFER FOLLOW-UP	Doctor:	'Is it OK if I see you again in a few days' time once you have thought things through?'
	Daughter:	*'Yes, thank you, Doctor. You've been very helpful, and I think that will allow me time to digest what you've told me today.'*
ELICIT FURTHER QUESTIONS AND CONCERNS	Doctor:	'Is there anything else I could help you with today before you go?'
	Daughter:	*'No. Thanks again for your help.'*

CONSULTATION END

CHAPTER 3

Cross-cultural communication

With the advent of modern communication systems and improved transport links, the world has been become a much smaller place. Large numbers of people are migrating from their birth places to other countries in pursuit of education, work and money. This has led some western countries to become a melting pot of culture and diversity. Consequently, the patient population which you, the doctor, will be required to treat and manage will be equally diverse. Within these populations there will exist a multitude of different beliefs, languages and cultures, each of which may act as a barrier in the doctor–patient relationship. You may be faced with problems in communication, misunderstandings, mistrust or even diametrically opposed ideals. You may at times feel uncomfortable or unnerved when dealing with such patients due to your ignorance about their beliefs and cultural practices.

However, as a doctor, your primary concern should be the welfare of the patient. You should not allow any personal prejudices to further burden an already difficult consultation. By educating yourself and exploring your own personal learning needs, you may be able to overcome these challenging hurdles. Reading and researching the cultural practices of the patients you are likely to encounter will not only make you a better clinician but also make you a well-rounded individual. Taking a little time in preparing and educating oneself in dealing with such patients may help to minimise misunderstandings and may improve the doctor–patient relationship.

Being aware of each and every cultural belief and practice is an impossible task. However, by utilising effective communication skills and adopting a simple framework, you will be able to adapt the consultation more effectively, acknowledging the patient's personal cultural beliefs, and negotiate treatment strategies around them.

In this chapter we describe some techniques that will help enhance your communications skills and give you an *aide-mémoire* to approach these difficult consultations. Towards the end of this chapter we have also provided a brief synopsis of the cultural beliefs and practices of the major world religions that may offer you useful insight into dealing with cross-cultural issues.

The importance of culture in communication

Culture may be defined as behaviours, practices and beliefs unique to a particular social, ethnic or religious group. Cultural practices are often formulated from an individual's family upbringing, religious affiliation, customary influences or as a by-product of the social environment they live in. Hence, the concept of culture should not be considered as something foreign or alien. Rather, each and every person can be identified with a particular culture and customary traditions.

If a person's beliefs and practices are different to one's own, feelings of awkwardness and embarrassment may be borne out during the consultation. You should appreciate that it is more than likely that the patient shares such feelings and is equally as uncomfortable in the situation as you are. Imagine if you became unwell in a foreign country and required urgent medical attention. The language and the environment will all appear unfamiliar to you. How difficult do you think it would be to express your symptoms, worries and fears to the receiving health professionals? You may harbour feelings of frustration and anguish at your own inability to communicate effectively and you may be confused by the medical advice being given. Many of the patients we see on a day-to-day basis have to struggle through this process all the time.

It is very easy to forget that no single culture is superior to another. Although you may feel that the practices of a particular patient may be strange and peculiar, this should not be allowed to impede your judgement about the patient nor their illness. Be careful not to impose your own cultural beliefs on the patient during the consultation. This will inevitably cause a clash of opinions and may turn the consultation sour.

Preparation

Admittedly, it is very difficult to be fully prepared to deal with people from all different types of backgrounds and cultures. However, there are commonalities in the way you can approach these patients.

It is worth taking time to look at the demographics of the area you are working in and identifying which cultural groups are prevalent. Try reading about their cultural practices, and perhaps contact the leaders of the local community to gain a better understanding of their values. Consider approaching staff members and fellow employees who are of a different background to your own. They can often be a valuable source of information regarding the different practices and expectations that patients of these cultures may have.

Pay particular attention to those beliefs which may directly affect medical management, such as religious periods of fasting and issues surrounding death. Be aware of the local services and links that you as the health professional have access to. Most hospitals have a chaplaincy that provides services for a wide range of religions and are readily available for help and advice.

Perhaps the biggest cultural barrier that can exist between the doctor and the patient is that of language. If the patient is unable to adequately express how they feel, they are likely to leave the consultation discontented and perhaps, more seriously, be misdiagnosed by the clinician.

Introducing yourself and establishing rapport

When introducing yourself to a patient of a different culture it is important to maintain your normal conduct as you would do with any other patient. You may appear insincere or even condescending if you were to change the way you speak or act towards the patient because of their background. It may even be brutally obvious to the patient that you are putting on a façade from your tactless approach. This would start the consultation off on the wrong foot, making the establishment of rapport virtually impossible thereafter.

Gender issues

Bear in mind that in some cultures it is not appropriate for a male to shake a female's hand or vice versa. In such situations, it may be more appropriate not to offer out your hand for shaking when greeting the patient. Rather, you should wait for the patient to make the first move and then reciprocate the gesture. In other cultures, patients of the opposite gender may insist on having a chaperone present in the room even if an intimate examination is not required. Do not take it to heart that this means the patient does not trust you. Instead, try to accommodate their request as best as you can with respect to the resources available to you. Female patients may feel more comfortable by bringing someone with them to the consultation. It may be interpreted as being impolite if you were to ask that individual to leave even if you were discussing sensitive matters.

Introductions

You should maintain the formality of the occasion by addressing the patient by their full name. In some cultures visiting the doctor is considered a formal event as the doctor is viewed as a 'ritual healer'. If you break with formality the patient may feel that you are belittling the seriousness of their illness.

Try not to feel too threatened by a name you cannot pronounce. The patient will probably appreciate that you have made a genuine attempt at pronouncing their name as opposed to addressing them with terms such as 'sir' or 'madam'. It is also worth bearing in mind that naming systems may vary from culture to culture. In some far-eastern cultures for example, the family name is placed before the forename. Asking the patient how they wish to be addressed may help you avoid such difficulties. Be careful at attempting to ask the patient their 'Christian' name as this can easily be misconstrued as being insensitive.

Non-verbal communication

Non-verbal forms of communication play a more important role when communicating with an individual from a different culture. Both parties may be feeling uncomfortable in the consultation and this may heighten their awareness of non-verbal cues. By maintaining an open posture and good eye contact, you will convey trust and warmth to the patient thus easing any early anxieties or tensions. A closed posture may be interpreted as being judgemental or prejudiced and can dissuade the patient from opening up. Some patients may have difficulty expressing their feelings due to limitations with their language, and giving them non-verbal encouragement, such as gesturing with your hands or nodding your head, may help them communicate more freely.

The patient's health beliefs

In many cultures doctors still practice medicine in a prescriptive, doctor-centred approach whereby the patient's health beliefs are not encouraged. Although using a patient-centred framework – whereby you ask the patient's ideas, concerns and expectations of their problem – may generate a bemused response, do not let this deter you. The patient's own health beliefs may give you an invaluable insight into their understanding of the illness in the context of their culture.

Discovering the patient's cultural beliefs

When trying to uncover the patient's ideas about their own illness, it is essential to relinquish any preconceived notions that you may already have about them. People who hold certain religious or cultural beliefs are all too often aware of these stereotypes and may lose trust and confidence in you if they think that you are harbouring them. Furthermore, it may well be the case that the patient's own beliefs are quite the opposite to the stereotypical ideas portrayed about them, and they may take offence. Take for example, the cultural practices of a 70-year-old Indian man who migrated to the UK 40 years ago. They are likely to be quite different to those held by his 18-year-old granddaughter who was born and brought up in the UK. Consider the following:

Doctor: 'Hello, Mrs Singh! How are you?'

Mrs Singh: 'I'm fine thanks. I've brought my husband today, is that OK? We recently got married.'

| Doctor: | 'Of course it's OK. Congratulations on your marriage. Did your parents arrange the marriage then?' |
| Mrs Singh: | 'No! We've known each other for quite a while now and decided on tying the knot a couple of months back.' |

In the above example, the doctor tried to use a preconceived stereotype about the patient to establish rapport. Unfortunately in this situation, the patient did not fit the mould and as result may have taken offence by the comment made. This may reflect badly on the doctor and is likely to impact negatively on the remainder of the consultation.

When approaching contentious religious subjects with patients, you should tread cautiously. Most people hold preconceived ideas that religious texts and instructions are quite rigid and dogmatic. This may lead you to tarnish a whole community with the same brush thinking that they hold identical views to one another. However, most of the major religions allow for a degree of interpretation and leniency around orders and rituals, particularly in the context of health. Another point to note is that within any given religion there may exist numerous schools of thought, denominations and sects, often holding varying and occasionally conflicting opinions about the same issue. For example, amongst most Christian denominations, receiving a blood transfusion is generally acceptable; the belief that it is prohibited is particular to Jehovah's Witnesses. Within Judaism, the Reformist school of thought permits the delaying of burial and the routine undertaking of post-mortem examinations, whereas for the Orthodox Jew, the opposite is true.

Note that you should attempt to explore the cultural ideas of the patient only if relevant to the consultation at hand. Inappropriately asking about a particular cultural belief may cause undue embarrassment. This may make the patient feel belittled and compelled to justify their beliefs to you. A better approach would be to wait for a cue from the patient before exploring that particular health belief:

Doctor:	'Good afternoon, Mr Odumbe. My name is Dr Morrison. How can I help you today?'
Mr Odumbe:	'The ENT surgeon has suggested my child have her tonsils removed . . .'
Doctor:	'Yes . . .' (*Doctor nods head encouragingly*)
Mr Odumbe:	'Well, the surgeon was mentioning to me about the risk of bleeding, and that my daughter might need a transfusion.'
Doctor:	'Yes, that's right. Whilst the operation is a relatively safe procedure, there is a small risk of bleeding immediate afterwards and sometimes a blood transfusion may become necessary.'

Mr Odumbe: 'Well you see, Doctor, that's why I've come to see you. My child cannot have a blood transfusion as we are Jehovah's Witnesses.'

Doctor: 'Ah, I see. Can you tell me a little bit more about your beliefs regarding blood transfusions?'

In the above example, the doctor started off by asking the patient an open question and encouraged them to share their ideas by using non-verbal cues. This approach allowed the patient to speak freely and feel comfortable enough to broach the subject of their personal beliefs with the doctor.

Uncovering the patient's agenda

Patients attend the doctor for a variety of reasons. More often than not the patient will have an agenda that they wish to discuss with you. Patients are often guided by their cultural or religious views which may play an influential role in shaping this agenda. On occasion, a situation may arise whereby the patient's cultural or religious beliefs are at odds with the predominant medical opinion. A patient, therefore, may consult with you to seek advice on this potential conflict and of ways to overcome it.

Patients are usually aware about the areas in which their religious beliefs contradict mainstream medical advice. However, to broach this as the main topic of discussion with the doctor, although extremely important, may also be acutely embarrassing for them. Regardless of your own opinion of their cultural belief, it is important to help the patient to air these views for a number of reasons, the most important of which may be that the patient has attended solely for this concern. If you were to dismiss it, or not even entertain it, this will leave the patient feeling that their needs have been unfulfilled. Secondly, this may entrench in the patient's mind that the medical establishment is prejudiced and bigoted and may deter the patient from seeking further medical help as necessary. Lastly, by not uncovering the patient's agenda you have missed an ideal opportunity to inform and educate the patient in regards to their particular health needs. Consider the following example:

Doctor: 'Hi, are you Jacob's dad? I am Dr Phillips. I am sorry to say your son passed away so soon after coming into hospital. As he died within 24 hours of admission, the Coroner states that we must perform a full post-mortem to find the cause of death. I am here to inform you that he will be taken for this shortly.'

Mr Horowitz: 'A post-mortem! I cannot allow it to take place as it is against my religion.'

Doctor:	'I appreciate your point of view, but these are the rules and everyone has to abide by them . . .'
Mr Horowitz:	'You will be hearing from my lawyers about this!'

When talking with the patient about their cultural beliefs, you should remember it may affect them deeply. Hence, you should try to approach the subject sensitively and in a way that makes the patient feel secure and settled in discussing them. This will also help defuse any potential anxieties or hostilities that may arise between the doctor and patient. Now revisit the previous scenario with these points considered.

Doctor:	'Hello, Mr Horowitz. Mr name is Dr Phillips, I was one of the doctors in the team looking after your son. The whole team has been shocked by the sudden nature of his death, and our thoughts are with you and your family at this very difficult time.'
Mr Horowitz:	'Thank you for your kind words, Doctor. I think we are all in a state of shock at the moment.'
Doctor:	'I understand. I can only offer my deepest condolences. If you would like somebody to talk to, perhaps a member of the nursing staff, they would be more than happy to discuss things with you. I appreciate that this is a very difficult time for you, but there is something pressing that I need to discuss with you.'
Mr Horowitz:	'Is everything OK, Doctor?'
Doctor:	'As your son died quite suddenly, we need to try to establish what may have been the cause of his death. In order to do this we need to carry out a post-mortem examination.'
Mr Horowitz:	'A post-mortem?! Don't you think my son has suffered enough?! I can't allow this?! I just can't allow you to do it!' *PAUSE*
Doctor:	'Mr Horowitz. I can see this is causing you some distress. Do you have any specific reservations about the post-mortem examination?'
Mr Horowitz:	'The thought of you cutting up my son is something I just can't take, but more importantly it is against my religion.'
Doctor:	'Would you like to tell me a little bit more about the religious issues involved.'
Mr Horowitz:	'We are members of the Jewish community and doing post-mortems is against our religion. Our faith teaches us

47

to undertake the burial as soon as possible. For this reason, any delay in the funeral is considered unacceptable. We just want our son to rest in peace.'

In this scenario the doctor started off by expressing his condolences to the patient's father and has clearly established a good rapport with him. This is paramount, as the doctor will be shortly discussing a sensitive matter with him. When the doctor mentioned the need for a post-mortem, it was quite clear the patient was uncomfortable with this notion. By remaining empathic and non-dismissive, the doctor managed to uncover the patient's religious belief and unravel their agenda. Despite the patient's objections, the doctor continued to be supportive and allowed the patient time to bring up all the issues and concerns he had in relation to the post-mortem exam.

Doctor's agenda

When you graduate from medical school having completed your medical degree, you will have to take the Hippocratic Oath. You agree to, amongst other things, 'practise and prescribe to the best of my ability for the good of my patients, and to try to avoid harming them', as well as swearing to 'keep the good of the patient as the highest priority'.

Many patient groups interpret these articles to mean that the doctor is obliged to be the patient's advocate in meeting all of their wants and demands. However, this is a clear over-simplification of the complex reality that a doctor has to face. As a trained and qualified doctor, your job is to present the medical opinion to the patient in relation to their symptoms and problems. You are further constrained by a duty of responsibility to codes and ethics laid down by higher medical bodies such as the GMC, DoH and the BMA. It is your job as a doctor to balance all of these influencing factors before giving medical advice that is appropriate to the patient, irrespective of whether they agree with it or not. The potential for conflict between the patient's agenda and the doctor's agenda is further compounded if the patient adheres to strict religious or cultural beliefs.

Although your instincts may tempt you to avoid getting into dispute with the patient by not fully declaring your agenda, it is important that you do not do this. By stating the harsh reality of the medical agenda you are at least giving the patient the chance to weigh up this advice in the context of their beliefs and allow them to make an informed choice. In addition, failing to mention the medical advice may bring into question your fitness to practise and leave you open to complaints and litigation if things were to go wrong. One, therefore, must tread a careful path and negotiate through this potential minefield.

On rare occasions, the doctor's agenda may have to supersede the patient's agenda regardless of cultural sensitivities. In the case of a child who was brought in following a high-impact traffic accident and whose parents are Jehovah's Witnesses, one would be obliged to inform the parents that an urgent blood transfusion is the only treatment option available. Although it is known that Jehovah's Witnesses do not accept blood transfusions, in this situation, saving the child's life is paramount and supersedes the parents' wishes.

Negotiation

You should now find yourself in a position whereby you have uncovered the patient's agenda and explained the medical agenda. Although there may be some commonality between the two agendas, occasionally you will find them to be in opposition. Your task then would be to negotiate with the patient, attempting to find some middle ground whereby you can both agree a shared management plan. Sometimes this may be the most difficult task to perform in the consultation. More often than not, your expected outcome pivots on the willingness of the patient to concede ground. However, by using effective communication techniques you may be better equipped to advise and influence the patient towards the medical opinion. Consider how you would manage the following example:

Doctor: 'What did you hope to gain by seeing me today?'

Mr Miah: 'Well, I was looking for a way to continue taking my diabetes medications whilst fasting at the same time. I don't want to compromise on my beliefs, Doctor, but at the same time I want to look after my health too.'

In this example, the patient has clearly set out his own agenda and has revealed the internal conflict between his religious obligations and his medical needs. As a doctor the response that you give now may directly affect the mood of the remainder of the consultation. If you act in a confrontational manner, paternalistic in your advice and dismissive of the patient's cultural belief, you are likely to disengage the patient and provoke a defensive and antagonistic response. On the other hand, you are likely to get a more receptive response if you were to be non-judgemental, encouraging and supportive in your approach. This will generate a feeling of trust and confidence in the patient and create an environment whereby they are more accepting of your advice. In the previous example a useful response to the patient's query to taking medication during his fast would be:

Doctor: 'I understand how important this month is for you and the significance it plays in your religion. However, I also understand the dilemma you find yourself in. On the one

	hand, fulfilling your obligation to the fast and on the other hand, taking medication to control your diabetes. What do you think the potential problems may be for you during the fast?'
Mr Miah:	'Well, at the moment I am taking my medication around 10 a.m. in the morning. But during the fast I am not able to do this as it will break my fast. I was also advised to have three regular meals and I can't see how I can do that whilst I am fasting.'
Doctor:	'Whilst it is important to take your medication regularly and on time, there is some flexibility as to when you can take them. Have you thought about taking your medication just before you start your fast at dawn and at sunset when you break it? Regarding your concern about having three regular meals, whilst it is valid, I believe that having two reasonably sized meals on either side of the fast as well as a small snack before you sleep should not cause your sugar levels to drop too low. What are your thoughts about this?'

As you can see from this approach, the patient's cultural belief is being respected and explored. The doctor is giving medical advice to the patient in a non-prescriptive way and is trying to suggest possible ways of dealing with their dilemma. By including the patient in the management plan you will be more likely to obtain a positive outcome.

In the event of a clash of agendas

Unfortunately, in real life you may experience occasions when it will be very difficult for you to fully accommodate the patient's agenda into a planned course of action. This may create a feeling of apprehension and unease between the doctor and the patient. In such situations, it is important to remain calm, non-confrontational and understanding in order to defuse any possible tension. Take for example the scenario of the Jewish family expressing their concerns about a post-mortem examination. Although the doctor should show empathy towards the patient's beliefs and recognise them, he or she must act in accordance with the law and advise the family that this examination is compulsory.

Doctor:	'I appreciate and fully understand your beliefs towards undertaking the post-mortem examination. I'm afraid that in cases of a sudden death, we are duty bound by law to establish the cause of death of your son.'

Mr Horowitz:	'I just can't bear the thought of my son being butchered.'
Doctor:	'I understand your concerns, Mr Horowitz. Unfortunately, this is a legal requirement. I have been present at similar examinations before, and can say that the pathologists are highly professional medical practitioners who will ensure that they maintain the honour and sanctity of your son whilst performing the examination. Perhaps I can have a word with the Coroner on your behalf to try to have this examination done as soon as possible so that the funeral of your son is not delayed any further?'
Mr Horowitz:	'Yes, I would appreciate that.'
Doctor:	'The hospital has close contacts with a Jewish Rabbi from a local synagogue, we can arrange for him to see you if you so wish?'
Mr Horowitz:	'I would like that actually. Thank you for all your help, Doctor.'

The doctor is legally obliged to inform the patient that this examination is compulsory and the matter is not up for negotiation. Nevertheless, the doctor has been accommodative towards the cultural and religious concerns raised by the patient. Doing so has helped reduce some of the family's anxieties and offered some reassurance that their son's body will be respected appropriately.

Giving advice on religious matters

When talking with the patient about religious and cultural matters it may be tempting for you, particularly if you are of the same religion or culture, to try to impress your own personal beliefs on them. You should be wary of falling into this trap since denominations of the same religion may have widely varying opinions. Also, not all patients have the same level of devoutness and some may be more lax in their implementation or interpretation of their religious scriptures than others.

On the other hand, it may be perfectly acceptable if you do have some insight into the patient's religion to impart this to them and assess their response. For example:

| *Ms Mahmood:* | 'I am really worried about my diabetes and my upcoming fast. I have been having a number of hypo's whilst taking my insulin but my religion obliges me to fast in this month of Ramadan.' |
| *Doctor:* | 'What we might need to do is monitor your sugar levels and reduce the insulin dose you are taking. It may be that |

the dosage of your insulin is too high, which is causing your glucose to fall very low.

'However, I have heard from other Muslims that during the fast it is permitted for you to break it on those days when you are feeling particularly unwell. Is that true?'

Liaising with religious chaplains

At this juncture it may be useful to seek the assistance of a religious chaplain to reinforce the advice you have given. Nowadays, most NHS hospitals have access to a wide array of chaplains of different faiths who are trained in giving religious opinion in complex health-related matters. They may be able to offer valuable assistance particularly in dealing with challenging patients. Not all patients will need their services as they may have their own community leaders whom they turn to for advice and direction. In such situations, if feasible, you could ask the patient to consult them and return to you at a later date to discuss the outcomes and the next steps.

Closing up

As you draw close to the end of the consultation you may feel that you have imparted a lot of information to the patient. In fact you may have challenged their personal beliefs and unsettled them, and whilst you may believe that you have successfully negotiated through a tricky situation, the patient may still be in disagreement with the position you hold.

By summarising back the key points of the consultation this will afford you some time to reflect upon the sensitive areas that you have broached and help you ensure that the patient has no misunderstandings of what has been discussed. When doing so you should ask them if they have any questions or if they wish to clarify any points.

Follow-up

If you have agreed to follow up the patient, try to give them a specific date and time for them to be seen. This will create a timeline for the patient to prepare themselves to see you again. They may wish to contact their local respected religious leaders, do some reading, or even meet with organisations or patient groups to aid them in their decision process.

You may also wish to use this time to carry out your own research about the topic at hand and perhaps even invite a religious leader to the next meeting, with the patient's consent. It may be handy if you have access to a patient information leaflet that discusses the religious matters in detail, to give to the patient before they depart.

Doctor: 'I know that this is a very difficult time for you, Mr Horowitz, and I would just like to summarise what we have talked about. In order to determine the cause of your son's death, it will be necessary to carry out a post-mortem. I appreciate that you are concerned that there will be a delay in performing the funeral and that you have other concerns regarding the post-mortem itself. For this reason I will try to speed things up as much as possible by speaking to the pathologist. I will also arrange for a local Rabbi to discuss the concerns you have regarding the post-mortem. Are you happy with this?'

Once you are both happy with the outcome, you should close the consultation and thank the patient.

BRIEF SYNOPSIS OF THE MAJOR WORLD RELIGIONS

Whilst it is difficult to know about all the different cultural systems, it is good practice to educate yourself regarding some of the common terms and principles held amongst the major religions. This may help you accommodate and negotiate some of the possible conflicts you might encounter in your professional life working in an ethnically diverse population.

Islam (religion of Muslims)

Islam is an Arabic word that literally translates to mean 'submission'. Muslims consider themselves to be submitters to God or 'Allah', the term used for God in Arabic. The central concept of Islam is the principle of 'Tawheed', or oneness of the Creator. Muslims believe that God is singular, having no partners or any children. The Islamic faith was brought by the final Prophet Muhammad to the Arabian Peninsula in 610 CE. The Islamic faith is a continuation of the Abrahamic faiths with Muslims believing in Moses, Abraham, Noah and Jesus along with other prophets. Muslims believe that Jesus was one of the mightiest prophets sent by God, born by a miraculous birth to Mary and that he spoke in his cradle.

Special considerations
Modesty
Muslims follow a strict code of modesty, and generally will prefer to be examined by clinicians of the same gender. If this is not possible it is likely that Muslim women may request for their husband or a male relative to be present during the examination. For intimate examinations, Muslims may flatly refuse to be seen by the opposite gender. Try to be accommodative to their request if possible. However, under certain circumstances Muslims may accept the examination to be performed if it is deemed to be an emergency. Some orthodox Muslims may not even make eye contact with members of the opposite sex. You should not take offence if you experience this.

Diet
Muslims are permitted to eat fish, dairy products and all fruit and vegetables. However, meat that is consumed has to be ritually slaughtered and this is known as Halal meat. Generally Muslims are able to eat Kosher meat as the animal is slaughtered in a similar manner. Alcohol and pork are strictly forbidden for consumption. However, some flexibility may exist for medicinal products that contain such ingredients.

Muslims abstain from food and drink from dawn to dusk in the month of Ramadan annually. Please read p. 55 for more details.

Prayer

Muslims pray five times a day, facing towards Mecca in Saudi Arabia. Times of prayer are before sunrise, midday, early afternoon, evening, and at night. On Fridays, Muslim males often perform a congregational prayer at midday. You may find that your patients are absent from the wards during these times. It is important for them to pray in a clean area and they may use a small prayer mat to ensure this. It may be helpful in the hospital setting to make them aware of the location of the multi-faith prayer room. Some Muslims may also offer voluntary prayers in between the compulsory ones. Prior to praying, Muslims need to perform ritual ablution (wudu) whereby they wash their hands, face, arms and feet with clean water.

Religious festivals

Ramadan is one of the five pillars of the Muslim faith and is held during the ninth month of the Islamic lunar calendar. During Ramadan, the Muslim will eat a full meal before sunrise, and then fast for the remainder of the day until sunset.

Fasting during Ramadan is expected of all healthy Muslims who have reached the age of puberty. Muslims who are elderly or sick may be exempt from fasting by paying a financial recompense to the poor instead.

Some Muslims interpret the fast as being the prevention of any substance from entering the body. Hence, they may not permit administration of anything through the mouth (PO), nose (intranasal), injection (IM, IV) or by suppository (PR). This has significant implications for compliance with routine medical treatments (e.g. insulin in diabetics), or when admitted to hospital for any other reason.

Muslims have two main festivals in the year: Eid-ul-Fitr (the festival of breaking the fast) is the celebration following the completion of Ramadan; and Eid-ul-Adha (the festival of sacrifice) following pilgrimage (Hajj). On both Eids, Muslims will congregate in the Mosque and offer prayers whilst visiting relatives. On Eid-ul-Adha, it is usual for Muslims to offer a sacrifice of an animal in imitation of the Prophet Abraham who was ordered to sacrifice his son to God.

As death approaches

In Islam, death is considered to be the progression of the soul from this life to the Hereafter. As death approaches, the family of the patient may want to sit besides them, reciting verses from the Holy Qur'an and praying for the patient. The family may request for an Imam to be present as well.

Last offices

When the patient has passed away, it is important that the body should not be washed nor the nails cut. The washing and preparation of the body should be left for the family or for Muslim funeral directors to perform. Usually they will tie the patient's feet together with a thread around the toes, and bandage the face in order to keep the mouth closed. Muslims are always buried and enquiring about cremation may be considered disrespectful. Burial before sunset is preferred. Muslims may oppose post-mortems, but there is usually no objection if this is required by law. Consult an Imam if necessary.

Key terms

Qur'an – The Islamic holy book, which Muslims believe was revealed to the Prophet Muhammad by God and contains His exact Words. They consider it to be miraculous in nature and inimitable. Muslims treat the Qur'an with great respect and can touch it only after performing ritual ablutions (wudu).

Hadith – A collection of teachings and sayings of the Prophet Muhammad. They complement and explain the teachings of the Qur'an.

Mosque – A Muslim centre of worship and religious instruction. Prayers are led by an Imam (religious leader).

Judaism (religion of Jews)

Judaism is derived from the Hebrew word 'Juda' and is considered to be one of the first monotheistic religions. Its beliefs are derived from the Torah (Old Testament) and Talmud. According to their religious text, Jews consider themselves to be the chosen people of God who act out His commands on Earth. Although Judaism was founded by Moses, Jews often trace themselves back to the Prophet Abraham and his covenant with God. Jews believe that you can be Jewish only if you are born to a Jewish mother. Although there are Reform Jews who permit conversions, in Orthodoxy this is not accepted.

Special considerations

Modesty

Similar to Islamic principles, Orthodox Jews deem it immodest to be touched by the opposite gender. Try to be as accommodating as possible. Orthodox male Jews may keep their heads covered with a small skull cap (Kippah) along with some parts of their limbs. You should seek permission before removing the cap before an examination.

Diet

Most Jews will request to eat only Kosher meat, which is meat slaughtered in a ritual manner. Although slaughtered in a similar way, Jews are unlikely to eat Halal foods as they are required to separate milk and meat produce at all times. Separate sets of utensils are used for the two types of food and a time lapse is observed between eating one and then the other. Pork is strictly forbidden for consumption and only fish with fins and scales can be eaten. Prawns and shellfish are also forbidden.

Prayer

Jews pray three times each day: morning, afternoon and evening. Men will always cover their heads with a skull cap whilst praying.

Religious festivals

The Jewish day of rest, Shabbat or Sabbath, begins just before sunset on Friday and ends after sunset on Saturday. Its traditional ceremonies and prayers involve the lighting of two candles and consuming some bread and wine, and are very important to many observant Jews. Jews are meant to avoid shopping, cooking and cleaning during the Sabbath and usually perform these duties before nightfall on Friday. Jews would prefer to avoid minor treatment on the Sabbath.

The Jewish New Year or Yom Kippur, is known as the Day of Atonement, which is spent in fasting from food and drink for 25 hours and avoiding washing and the wearing of perfume. It is the most sacred day in the Jewish calendar as it is considered the day on which God prepares the destiny for an individual for the forthcoming year.

Succoth is the Jewish day of harvest and is celebrated five days after Yom Kippur. It is also known as the feast of Tabernacles and remembers the many years that the Jews spent in the wilderness at the time of Moses.

Pesach, or Passover, is the day of celebration remembering the salvation of the Jews from Egypt. Jewish people often eat a symbolic meal on this day consisting of unleavened bread, egg and salt water, bone of lamb and four cups of wine.

As death approaches

A dying patient may wish to make a deathbed confession, or recite the Hebrew Shema. They also may request for a Rabbi to be present. In Jewish tradition it is best not to leave the dying patient alone.

Last offices
A Rabbi should be contacted immediately when the patient passes away. The body should be covered in a plain white sheet and relatives may wish to keep a vigil by the body. Jews are buried and this should take place as soon as possible after death. Post-mortem examinations are not permitted unless the Coroner requests this. For further information consult a Rabbi if this is required.

Key terms
Synagogue – The Jewish place of worship.

Rabbi – Religious leader at the synagogue. Some Jewish families may seek advice from their own Rabbi about issues relating to the patient's treatment.

Torah – The main Jewish holy book (the first five books of the Christian Old Testament).

Tallith – Prayer shawl worn by men for morning prayers.

Jehovah's Witnesses
Jehovah's Witness is a Christian religious movement that was founded in the late nineteenth century in America by Charles Taze Russell. Jehovah's Witnesses consider the Bible to be the only authority for their beliefs and practices and tend to take the literal interpretation of the text. They are known to refuse blood transfusions as they interpret the following text to indicate this: *'to keep abstaining from things sacrificed to idols and from blood and from things strangled and from fornication.'* (Acts 15)

Special considerations
Modesty
Any sexual relationship outside marriage is a grave sin and can cause the person to leave the fellowship. Abortion is considered a great crime and indeed tantamount to murder. Members are forbidden from smoking, using recreational drugs and gambling.

Blood transfusions
Jehovah's Witnesses believe that a human being may not sustain their life with the blood of another person. This belief is firmly held, and the patient is likely to refuse a blood transfusion even if this means risking death. Many Jehovah's Witnesses carry advance directives requesting that medical staff do not use blood or blood products as a form of treatment. Most Jehovah's Witnesses are well informed about their religious teaching, and about their legal right

to refuse treatment. Most Jehovah's Witness parents will refuse transfusions for their children. In extreme circumstances a court order may be required to overrule the beliefs of the family.

Blood tests
Blood is seen to represent life itself and thus specimens must be treated with respect, and disposed of with care.

Organ transplant
Some Jehovah's Witnesses may refuse to receive an organ due to the transplanted organ containing residual blood.

Diet
Jehovah's Witnesses will refrain from eating meat with residual blood. Therefore, animals are usually bled after slaughter. To err on the side of caution, some Jehovah's Witnesses prefer to be vegetarian. Jehovah's Witnesses, unlike followers of Judaism or Islam, can consume pork if it is slaughtered and bled correctly.

Festivals
Jehovah's Witnesses do not respect Sunday as a holy day, nor do they celebrate Christmas, Easter or birthdays. Their most important and solemn event is the celebration of the 'Lord's Evening Meal', or the 'Memorial of Christ's Death'.

Prayer
Jehovah's Witnesses meet and perform prayer in Kingdom Halls. They usually attend weekly, and these meetings are used to study the Bible and associated doctrines. They may also sing hymns and offer brief prayers as worship.

As death approaches
A dying patient may receive a number of visitors as congregational support is important. Although there are no formal religious rites when a person is dying, quiet prayer with a local Elder may be appreciated.

Last offices
Last offices are performed as normal, unless the family have special wishes. The body should be wrapped in a plain sheet. There is no religious prohibition against post-mortem, but most Jehovah's Witnesses refuse them if there is no legal requirement. They may be cremated or buried depending on the patient's or family's preference.

Key terms

Kingdom Hall – The place where the local Jehovah's Witness fellowship assembly meets.

Hinduism (religion of Hindus)

Hinduism is an umbrella term covering the predominant religions in the Indian subcontinent. It is one of the oldest world religions, however it does not have a recognised central religious text or a single founder. The term Hindu is derived from the name of the river Indus, which passes from Tibet into Pakistan. Although Hindus believe in a central God figure known as Vishnu, most worship associated partners such as Durga, Krishna, Shiva, Ganesha, Hanuman, Kali, Murugan, Venkateshwara, Nataraja, Rama, and Lakshmi.

Special considerations
Modesty

Hindu women can be very reluctant to undress for examination and will prefer to be examined by other females. Discomfort or pain in the genitor-urinary or bowel areas is often seen as a taboo subject. Patients will not volunteer information of symptoms in these body systems, especially if a spouse is present.

Hygiene

Hindus need running water (or a jug of water) in the same room as a toilet, which they use to clean themselves. A bowl of water should be offered after a bedpan. Showers are preferred to baths as they provide a source of running water.

Diet

Beef is forbidden for Hindus as cows are considered sacred creatures. Many Hindus are vegetarian. They may prefer to use plates that have been used only for vegetarian food. Some are vegan and do not eat eggs or dairy products.

Fasting

During special festivals such as Diwali, some Hindus may fast on certain days. Each October on Karva Chot, many Hindu women abstain from food from dawn to night. On occasions, some Hindu women chose to fast on Tuesdays while men fast on Saturdays.

Prayer

Hindus generally pray twice daily and their worship involves chanting mantras, a form of vibrational sound. The chanting of mantras is the most popular form of worship in Hinduism. Yoga and meditation are also considered as a form of devotional service towards their deity.

As death approaches

Hindus consider the soul as an eternal being which passes through this life encapsulated in a physical body. When a person dies, their soul is believed to continue to exist and reincarnated into another physical form before finally attaining its rest in eternal liberation. For this reason, death is not seen as a final calamity but rather an ongoing continual process in the search of tranquillity.

Hindu patients would prefer to die at home, where they have their own shrine. Death in hospital can be extremely distressing for Hindu relatives, who must be called immediately if death is felt to be imminent. When death is considered inevitable, the Pandit, a Hindu teacher, may come to the hospital to pray with the relatives of the dying patient. The last rites, or 'puja', may be performed by the priest or by the family. They may wish to use lamps, candles or incense as part of the ritual. The priest may tie a thread around the neck or wrist of the patient, and it should not be removed.

Last offices

The family may wish to perform the last offices in hospital. If so, they will wash the deceased in water mixed with drops from the Ganges River. Hindus are always cremated and next-day cremation is preferred. Death and cremation certificates should be provided with the least possible delay. Hindus generally do not take exception to post-mortem examinations, especially if required by law.

Key terms

Karma – Hindu doctrine, which teaches that every action somebody does in this life will affect them in the next.

Dharma – Freeing the soul from the cycle of death and rebirth by living a good and virtuous life.

Brahmin – The highest Hindu caste from which the Pandit (priest) is chosen.

Harijan – The lowest Hindu caste (untouchables); some Hindus still hold firm to the caste system and are not allowed to marry outside their caste.

Mandir – Hindu temple.

Vedas – A collection of the holiest books in Hinduism.

FIRST CLINICAL SCENARIO

Orthodox Jew and autopsy

You may be faced with a situation where you must discuss management plans that are at odds with the beliefs or cultural practices of the patient or their relatives. When informing the family of this, you should try to be tactful in your approach whilst remaining sensitive to their cultural beliefs. However, there may be occasions where room for manoeuvre is restricted. Your plan of action must be made clear, even if it goes against the wishes of the patient or relatives.

Although it is common courtesy to keep the family informed about their relative's progress, their personal opinions or wishes cannot necessarily over-rule medical decisions.

DOCTOR'S BRIEF

You are the Foundation House Officer in ITU. Joseph is an 18-year-old student who has been in the department for a week following a serious road traffic accident. During this time, he has remained unconscious on a ventilator. Following extensive investigation, discussions, and a diagnosis of brainstem death by the neurologists, your team has decided that the ventilator should be switched off, as there is no realistic prospect of the patient coming out of a coma. Joseph's father, an Orthodox Jew, has come into the department and you have been asked by the nurse-in-charge to explain the decision. You have been told that the father is fully aware that his son's injuries are very serious, that his condition is critical, and that he is unlikely to survive.

ACTOR'S BRIEF *(if you are the doctor, please do not read)*

You are Mr Haslam, Joseph's father. Although the initial news of the accident came as a shock to you, you are fully aware that your son's condition is critical. As each day passes with your son on the ventilator, your hopes fade of a recovery and you are now prepared for the worst.

However, you have not lost all hope and whilst your son is still breathing and has a heartbeat you continue to pray for his survival. You are an Orthodox Jew and you have a strong desire to ensure that everything possible is being done to keep your son alive. As far as you are concerned, your son is still alive and all efforts to keep him that way must continue.

Although you are prepared for his likely death, you will not accept he has died until his heart stops beating of its own accord.

SCENARIO WALK-THROUGH

INTRODUCE YOURSELF TO THE PATIENT'S RELATIVE AND ESTABLISH RAPPORT	*Doctor:*	'Hello, Mr Haslam. My name is Dr Gorman. I was wondering if I could have a word about your son's progress?'
	Mr Haslam:	*'Yes, of course, Doctor.'*
	Doctor:	'It's a little noisy on the ward, do you think that it might be better if we went to a quieter place?'
	Mr Haslam:	*'Yes. That would be fine . . .'*

IN THE RELATIVES' ROOM

OPEN QUESTION	*Doctor:*	'Mr Haslam, how do you feel things have progressed in regards to your son's health?'
	Mr Haslam:	*'To be honest, I think you have all done such a fantastic job. I know he is not well, but you never know, miracles do happen.'*
ESTABLISH RELATIVE'S IDEAS	*Doctor:*	'Yes. He was quite unstable on admission. What do you think of his current condition?'
	Mr Haslam:	*'Well, I know that he has been in a critical condition whilst he has been in here. It's been quite difficult to come to terms with, especially when I saw some doctors who examined him and they told me that parts of his brain had "switched off". He's my only boy and I love him so much.'*
ESTABLISH RELATIVE'S CONCERNS	*Doctor:*	'Is there anything in particular you are worried about?'
DEMONSTRATE ACTIVE LISTENING (EYE CONTACT, OPEN BODY POSTURE)	*Mr Haslam:*	*'Look, I know he might not make it. I have heard rumours that sometimes with old people they switch off the life-support machine. I hope that you won't do that with my young son.'*
SIGNPOSTING DIFFICULT NEWS TO FOLLOW	*Doctor:*	'Mr Haslam, I do have something quite important to discuss with you about your son's treatment.'
	Mr Haslam:	*'Is everything OK, Doctor?'*
	Doctor:	'As you said, two of our specialist doctors recently examined your son and determined that important areas of his brain that control his breathing have stopped working. This is why he is on a ventilator machine – he is unable to breathe on his own. This is known as "brainstem death".'

USE OF PAUSES	

PAUSE

Mr Haslam: *'Yes, the other doctors informed me about this too . . .'*

GIVE THE INFORMATION IN CLEAR, UNAMBIGUOUS LANGUAGE	

Doctor: 'As these vital parts of the brain are no longer functioning, we as a team feel that the ventilator is no longer fulfilling its purpose.

PAUSE

'We have come to the difficult decision that we will have to withdraw the ventilator support.'

PAUSE

Mr Haslam: *'I'm afraid I can't allow you to do that.'*

PAUSE

EXPLORE CONCERNS AND BELIEFS	

Doctor: 'I understand it may be difficult decision for you to accept. Is there anything in particular that you would like to discuss . . .?'

RELATIVE'S CULTURAL AGENDA	

Mr Haslam (emotionally): *'Well . . . as Orthodox Jews, we don't recognise this idea of brainstem death. So long as he is breathing and his heart is working, as far as I am concerned he is alive. I know that medically you say these functions are not working, but in such a situation, I must abide by what is correct in my religion. I forbid you from switching the machine off. That is my final decision.'*

PAUSE

SHOW EMPATHY AND MANAGE RELATIVE'S EMOTIONAL RESPONSE	

Doctor: 'I appreciate this is a very difficult time for you . . . I respect your religious views about this matter. However, I must inform you that the decision to withdraw the ventilator support can only be made on clinical grounds and on the likelihood of survival.'

Mr Haslam: *'Well, you're telling me, in effect, that you're pulling the plug on my son, and doing something against my religion.'*

Doctor: 'I think it's important to point out that the ventilator is simply performing some of the vital functions for him, as he not able to carry these out for himself anymore. When we do switch off the machine, your son will pass away peacefully.'

Mr Haslam: *'But how can you ask me to commit such a grave sin, and that too, on my own son?'*

EXPLORE RELIGIOUS/ CULTURAL BELIEFS	*Doctor:*	'In no way do we intend for you to commit a sin. These decisions are made on clinical grounds by the doctors and we bear full responsibility for them.
	PAUSE	
		'I am sorry to have had to give you this news. It may be an idea if you discuss this with a religious leader from your community.'
	Mr Haslam:	*'I remember being told by someone that we recognise death only as a natural process. By switching off the machine, are we not playing the role of God? But I haven't had the chance to discuss it with my Rabbi yet. Things have happened just so quickly.'*
OFFER APPROPRIATE SUPPORT (RELIGIOUS/ CULTURAL)	*Doctor:*	'I can see that this is a very complex matter and is not straightforward. If you wish, we can put you in touch with one of our Jewish chaplains, who are very experienced in dealing with these sorts of situations?'
	PAUSE	
	Mr Haslam:	*'OK, I think that might be quite useful.'*
	Doctor:	'Well, we will try to arrange that quite urgently. I think that you will find it helpful to talk all this through with someone who can see things from both the medical and religious perspectives.'
	Mr Haslam:	*'That's fine. Do let me know when you can put me in touch with them.'*
SUMMARISE BACK	*Doctor:*	'Yes, I will do so, definitely. Before we conclude can I just go over some of the things we discussed?'
	Mr Haslam:	*'Yes, OK.'*
	Doctor:	'Unfortunately, your son suffered severe brain injury as the result of a car accident and is no longer able to breathe independently. We have come to the conclusion that your son is too unwell ever to breathe on his own and the ventilator regrettably will not improve his chances of survival.
	PAUSE	
		'Our team has arrived at a difficult decision to withdraw the ventilator support. This of course must be difficult to hear and we take on board your reasons for wanting it to continue.

PAUSE

'I appreciate your religious concerns and for this reason will be arranging for the Jewish chaplain to discuss this matter with you urgently.

PAUSE

'Are you happy with this?'

Mr Haslam: 'Yes, Doctor.'

CHECK RELATIVE'S
UNDERSTANDING OF
INFORMATION GIVEN

Doctor: 'Is there anything you wish me to clarify or go through again with you?'

Mr Haslam: 'No, thank you, Doctor.'

ELICIT FURTHER
QUESTIONS AND
CONCERNS

Doctor: 'Do you have any other questions you wish to ask?'

Mr Haslam: 'No, thank you. I think I need some time by myself.'

Doctor: 'I am happy to see you after you have talked things through with the Rabbi. Is that OK?'

Mr Haslam: 'Yes. Thank you.'

CONSULTATION END

SECOND CLINICAL SCENARIO

Catholic considers abortion

When dealing with religious issues you should be sensitive and considerate in your approach. Be careful of judging the patient and avoid giving any religious advice or counsel. Instead, you should adopt a neutral position and allow the patient time to make an informed choice. Direct them, if necessary, to a chaplain who is better placed to give them religious direction and advice.

DOCTOR'S BRIEF

You are Dr Singh, a Foundation Year doctor undertaking your placement in General Practice. Ms O'Leary is a 26-year-old project manager who has come to the surgery today.

ACTOR'S BRIEF *(if you are the doctor, please do not read)*

You are Caroline O'Leary, a 26-year-old single woman born and brought up in Cork, Ireland. You recently moved to the UK and you are a successful project manager. You have always been a devout Catholic, and you attend church every Sunday and midweek. Recently, you were on a business trip, and after a hard day you went to the pub. You met someone whilst you were there, which ended in a one-night stand. You have had no contact with this person since.

You have found out recently that you are pregnant and you are very confused as to whether or not you want to continue with the pregnancy. Your reason for wanting a termination is to cover up your sin of premarital relationship and avoid social exclusion. However, you also feel that 'two wrongs don't make a right'. You are quite nervous, and need lots of encouragement to talk about this.

If you feel that the doctor is coming across as judgemental then you will refuse to answer any probing questions.

SCENARIO WALK-THROUGH

INTRODUCE YOURSELF TO THE PATIENT AND ESTABLISH RAPPORT	*Doctor:*	'Hello, Ms O'Leary. My name is Dr Singh. How are you today?'
	Ms O'Leary:	*'Erm . . . Not too bad, Doctor. Things have been quite difficult recently.'*
OBSERVE PATIENT FOR NON-VERBAL CUES	*Doctor:*	'You seem a little uneasy. Is there anything in particular that you would like to discuss with me today?'
	Ms O'Leary:	*'Really, Doctor, I don't know where to start . . .'* (Patient remains silent)
ENCOURAGE THE GUARDED PATIENT TO ELICIT CONCERNS	*Doctor:*	'Don't worry. You have obviously made the effort to come and seek advice. Everything that you mention to me today is held in strict confidence and will remain private.'
	Ms O'Leary:	*'The thing is, I did a pregnancy test a few days back, and I found out that I was pregnant . . .'*
	PAUSE	
NON-JUDGEMENTAL WITH SENSITIVE INFORMATION	*Doctor:*	'OK . . . and how did that make you feel?'
	Ms O'Leary:	*'I know this sounds terrible, but for me it's the worst possible news . . .'*
OPEN QUESTIONING, ESTABLISH PATIENT'S AGENDA	*Doctor:*	'In what way is this bad news for you?'
	Ms O'Leary:	*'In every way possible, Doctor!'*
	PAUSE	
SHOW EMPATHY	*Doctor:*	'I am here to offer you help and support, whatever the circumstances may be. It would be helpful if you could tell me about some of the difficulties you have been experiencing.'
	Ms O'Leary:	*'First of all, the father is someone I do not really know very well. I met him at the pub after a difficult day whilst on a business trip, and one thing led to another. I haven't really seen him since. He doesn't even know.'*
NON-VERBAL CUES TO ENCOURAGE PATIENT TO TALK	*Doctor:*	'I see . . .'
	Ms O'Leary:	*'Obviously that's bad enough, but the thing is, Doctor, I am, or I guess I should say I was, a devout Catholic. Having sex outside of wedlock is forbidden for me. I guess in the eyes of God, I have committed an unforgivable sin.'*

	Doctor:	'Have you spoken to anybody about this?'
CHECK FOR SUPPORT NETWORKS	Ms O'Leary:	'NO! That's the last thing I could possibly do, Doctor! If this gets out into the local church community . . . my parents would probably disown me . . .'
ESTABLISH PATIENT'S EXPECTATIONS	Doctor:	'Have you thought about what you might want to do from here?'
	Ms O'Leary:	'I only have one option, Doctor . . . I need to have an abortion . . .'

PAUSE

AFFIRM YOUR ROLE TO THE PATIENT	Doctor:	'Ms O'Leary, I appreciate it was difficult for you to mention all this to me. The decision as to whether you want to continue with the pregnancy or terminate, is one which ultimately you will have to make. I am here though to try to offer you support with whatever you decide.'
	Ms O'Leary:	'Doctor, I'm just so confused.'
OPEN QUESTION	Doctor:	'What's confusing you?'
	Ms O'Leary:	'I know I have sinned, Doctor. But I don't know whether I should continue with this pregnancy and live with the open shame of my sin, or whether I should terminate and commit another sin. I can hide from my community but I can't hide from the Lord.'

PAUSE

	Doctor:	'I can see the difficult dilemma you are in. Perhaps it may be worth trying to talk through these issues with someone before you come to your final decision about what you want to do with the pregnancy. Would you agree with that?'
	Ms O'Leary:	'I just feel so confused right now. One minute I think I need to have an abortion, the next, I think two wrongs don't make a right . . .'
	Doctor:	'How would you feel about speaking to a priest about your difficulties?'
	Ms O'Leary:	'No, Doctor! I couldn't possibly risk the prospect of this getting out.'
OFFER APPROPRIATE SUPPORT (RELIGIOUS/ CULTURAL)	Doctor:	'Well, you could speak to one of the Catholic chaplains who is attached to the local hospital, perhaps? We have a few contacts we could put you in touch with.

		Not only are they well versed in the religious aspects of patient care, but also they are highly trained and you can certainly approach them in the strictest confidence.'
	Ms O'Leary:	'I guess it is something I could consider.'
	Doctor:	'You may also wish to see our counsellor who will be able to support you through this difficult time.'
	Ms O'Leary:	'Yes, Doctor. I think that might help to sort out this confusion . . .'
ARRANGE FOLLOW-UP	Doctor:	'I am always here to offer whatever advice I can. Why don't you make an appointment to see me in two weeks' time after you have talked things through with a priest? If you feel you need to see me more urgently, then do get in touch with the practice and I'll see what I can do.'
	Ms O'Leary:	'Thanks, Doctor. I'll get in touch with those contacts you have provided me with.'

CONSULTATION END

CHAPTER 4

Communicating with an angry patient

Anger is one of the most intense emotions that can be expressed by human beings. We all get angry from time to time for various reasons. However, not everyone has the self-control to manage this emotion appropriately. Lack of control over an individual's anger may allow it to escalate and translate into verbal or physical violence. Such behaviour, in the healthcare setting, should never be tolerated regardless of who the perpetrator is or their reasons.

In today's society, with the advent of the '24-hour' culture, people's wants and expectations have become more demanding. Some individuals may insist on being seen and treated instantly, regardless of their actual medical need. Others may be disproportionately fearful of their symptoms and request to be seen out of turn. To compound all of this, the stresses of illness can cause emotions to be heightened and lead to patients displaying anger, especially when things do not go in their favour. This may create a volatile situation that has the ability to become unsavoury. They way you go about managing this predicament has a huge bearing on its final outcome.

Dealing with an angry patient

One of the main challenges doctors face when communicating with an aggressive patient is to calm them down sufficiently such that they are open to reason and dialogue. Patients often display anger in order to bring attention to an injustice they have experienced, or simply to express their frustrations. In most cases, they do not set out or plan to become troublesome or violent. However, when provoked or antagonised, violence may ensue.

Your intention, in such situations, should be to reduce the threat of harm to yourself and others. This can be achieved by employing simple techniques and strategies that will help to calm the patient down.

Communication strategies

The greatest mistake you can make when confronting an angry patient is to reciprocate anger with anger. In the heat of the moment, you may be inclined to shout at the patient, use swear words and expletives, or simply interrupt and talk over them when they are speaking. Such behaviour will fan the flames of anger and only infuriate them further. By saying a few calm words, adopting a relaxed posture and being empathic, you should be able to settle the angriest of patients and defuse the situation.

Body language

When a person becomes angry they often assume facial expressions and postures that convey aggression and hostility. They may stand bolt upright with tense, lowered eyelids and a staring gaze, pointing in an accusatory manner. As a doctor you should be careful to avoid defensively mimicking their body language, and instead employ body language that conveys amity and understanding. Adopt an open, relaxed posture that is calm and inviting. Avoid invading the patient's own personal space and making prolonged eye contact. Ensure that your hands are kept out of your pockets and remain open. Keep your arms uncrossed and hold your head at a slight angle. This will make you appear less threatening and more receptive to the patient's problems.

Speed and tone of voice

An aggressive patient may speak with a loud voice and harsh tone, bellowing their demands to others. By speaking in a gentle, calm and soft manner, you may be able to win over the patient and appease them.

Active listening

As we have mentioned, patients become angry in order to communicate their demands and frustrations. Being dismissive and incessantly interrupting them is likely to incense them further. It is better to demonstrate active listening and permit the patient to vent their anger. This often has the effect of calming them down as they feel that they have been listened to.

Empathic approach

Angry patients may feel that their concerns are being dismissed and not attended to. They may have already encountered staff members who have not been sympathetic to their plight. Hence, when speaking to the patient you should try to demonstrate empathy. This will show that you value their concerns and wish to act in their best interests. Try to show the patient that you are actually hearing what they say, and understand how they feel. Take their concerns seriously, even if they appear to be misplaced.

The consultation: the angry patient

No one likes to deal with an angry patient, for fear of making the situation worse. A hostile patient can pose a number of dangers and difficulties to yourself and those around you. However, with a well thought-out framework and plan, taking into account some of the principles outlined above, you should be able to defuse and manage most of the difficult scenarios you may encounter.

Preparation

It is vital that you try to ascertain from your colleagues or nursing staff why the patient is angry, before you go and see them. Background information such as whether the patient has learning difficulties, has an acute emergency or is under the influence of intoxicants, may affect how you manage the situation. Gather as much information as possible, as the patient will feel more frustrated if you appear ignorant about their condition and the treatment they have received thus far.

Privacy

After arming yourself with enough information to approach the patient, try to draw them away from any crowded seating areas or public places. It may be a good idea to take them to a side room so that any ensuing conversations are kept private and confidentiality is maintained. This may not only reduce the risk of creating a spectacle for others, but will also help focus the conversation back onto the patient's grievances.

Safety

If you suspect that the patient may become violent and that your personal safety could be compromised, it is important to prepare yourself and your surroundings for this possibility. Remove any unnecessary items from the side room so that it does not contain anything that could be used as a missile or weapon. Keep seating to a minimum and place your seat nearer the door to allow a quick exit if need be. Inform other staff of your intentions to meet the patient and the location of the consultation. Carry a panic alarm or bring a colleague with you if you consider the threat of violence to be genuine.

Introducing yourself and establishing rapport

Introduce yourself clearly and state your role. An angry patient will want to know who you are and how you can help them. Make an attempt to establish rapport even though they may be dismissive of your initial efforts. When communication is difficult, the patient may not want to engage in meaningful conversation straight away. However, persistence in trying to build rapport may eventually bear fruit as you slog your way through the consultation.

It may be easy to charge into the encounter, accusing the patient of making a scene, without establishing the underlying reasons for their grievances. This may generate a knee-jerk reaction from the patient, causing them to immediately disengage and become more hostile. Consider the following example:

Patient:	*(BELLOWING)* 'I demand to see a doctor!'
Doctor:	*(SHOUTS BACK)* 'I am sorry sir. You have to wait your turn like everyone else!'
Patient:	'Who are you? What do you want?'
Doctor:	'That's not important. We have a zero-tolerance policy for behaviour like yours. Since you have come here you have created a scene and upset most of the staff.'
Patient:	'If you doctors bothered to do your job properly instead of chatting all day then maybe some of us would be seen earlier!'
Doctor:	'I don't like the tone of your voice! You have to wait your turn patiently like everyone else or get out!'

In the example above, the doctor reacted to the patient's provocation by being confrontational and dismissive. This infuriated the patient further and turned the consultation into a slanging match. A better way would be to placate the patient by making disarming statements that signify your intentions to be helpful.

Patient:	*(BELLOWING)* 'I demand to see a doctor!'
Doctor:	'Hello, Mr Smith. I am Dr Mitchell, one of the A&E doctors.'
Patient:	'I don't want to see you. I want to see your boss, now!'
Doctor:	'Well, unfortunately they are not available right now but I am here to help in anyway I can.'
Patient:	'Your staff are useless and I want to make an official complaint!'
Doctor:	'I understand you are upset. Can we go somewhere more private to discuss this?'

Understanding the patient's perspective

Patients may become aggrieved due to unaddressed frustrations that have been left to simmer. These emotions may boil over when they feel that they have been treated unfairly in some way. By trying to appreciate the patient's point of view you may be able to rationalise their behaviour and offer immediate practical solutions that can redress some of their aggravation.

Establish the reasons for their behaviour

Start off by asking a simple open question such as, *'What seems to be the problem?'* Give ample space and time for them to vent their anger, and allow them to do most of the talking. This will go some way towards calming them down and making them open to reason.

Make sure you demonstrate active listening to show the patient that you are actually interested in what they are saying. Express empathy and concern and apologise for any distress caused.

Doctor:	'Hello, Mr Lewis. My name is Dr Daniel. How are you today?'
Mr Lewis:	*(Says angrily)* 'How do you think I am, eh?!'
Doctor:	'Mr Lewis, something seems to be troubling you . . . would you like to . . .'
Mr Lewis:	'TROUBLING ME! Is that all you can say? TROUBLING ME!
	SILENCE
	(SHOUTING) 'Do you know how long I've been waiting here? I've been more than five hours pal! Now you tell me . . . what do you think is troubling me?
	SILENCE
	'I can't walk, I've been sitting in this waiting room waiting for an X-ray for years . . . and all you people seem to be doing is just rushing off and ignoring me! I'm in pain!'
Doctor:	*(Says empathically)* 'I am really sorry that you had to wait so long. You must be in a lot of pain . . .'

Acknowledgement of the patient's emotional state

It is important to demonstrate to the patient that you have acknowledged the fact that they are upset and angry and that you empathise with their situation. This will show them that you appreciate the magnitude of their problem and will, hopefully, reinforce the idea that you are there to help.

Consider the following example of a patient who has been told that their operation has been cancelled and that it will be rebooked for another day:

Doctor:	'I'm afraid your operation has been cancelled.'
Patient:	'What? That's the third time!'
Doctor:	'Yes. I'm afraid the Consultant is away on holiday. We will rebook it in due course.'
Patient:	'I don't believe it! What do we pay our taxes for? This is outrageous!'
Doctor:	'Yes, quite. How unfortunate. Anyway, you will be getting an appointment in the post. Goodbye for now.'

Patient: 'This is a disgrace! An absolute disgrace!'

Now consider how the doctor could have handled the situation differently:

Doctor: 'I'm afraid your operation has been cancelled.'

Patient: 'What? That's the third time!'

Doctor: 'I'm very sorry, Mr Owen. I really am.'
    PAUSE

Patient: 'This is an absolute outrage!'
    SILENCE

Doctor: 'I can see you're very upset about this.'

Patient: 'Upset? I'm absolutely livid that you could do this to me again!'
    SILENCE

Doctor: 'I know it must be incredibly frustrating and I fully appreciate that you feel angry about this. I really am sorry.'

Patient: 'It's alright for you!'

Doctor: 'Obviously I'm not in your position. But I am sure that if I was, I would feel just as upset as you are. However, unfortunately these things do sometimes happen – and it is very unfortunate that this is the third time it has happened to you.'

Patient: 'Look, I know it's not your fault. But I'm just fed up at having to wait so long to get my knee sorted . . .'

The doctor has, in the example above, demonstrated that he appreciates the patient's emotional state and has attempted to empathise with him. He has also made good use of appropriate silences and pauses to allow the patient to vent his anger and subsequently cool down. Whilst this may not solve the situation, it will at the very least, go some way towards appeasing the patient, calm him down and preventing things from getting out of hand.

Offer an explanation

A patient may become angry due to a failing in the system or how they have been dealt with. They may be oblivious to the pressure and demands that medical staff are constantly under, which may have contributed to the failings. Hence, a simple explanation as to what the circumstances are may reduce much of their frustration.

Mr Lewis: 'Do you know that I have been waiting patiently in agony for four hours? Whilst I have been here I've seen at least three people who came after me, go in and be seen before me! How is that fair?!'

Doctor:	'I am sorry that you have had to wait for so long in pain. This is unacceptable. Unfortunately, it has been a particularly busy shift today. Normally in casualty, we prioritise patients the moment they come in. We try to see those patients who need medical treatment most urgently, first. Unfortunately, today we have had an unexpectedly large number of cases like that, and that's why you have had to wait.'

Establish what the patient wants and offer solutions

Having established possible explanations as to why the patient is angry, you should now proceed to find out what the patient actually wants. They might want something simple, such as painkillers, which is not unreasonable and can easily be addressed. On the other hand, their demands may be completely impractical, excessive and not deliverable without being unfair to others. In both cases, make a sincere attempt to negotiate with the patient and offer realistic solutions to their problems.

Mr Lewis:	'I didn't know that. That seems entirely fair. However that does not give me any relief for my pain.'
Doctor:	'I am sorry that you have been left in pain for so long. I will make sure that you get some painkillers before you are seen by a casualty doctor.'
Mr Lewis:	'I've been waiting for so long, I don't know if I have broken something. It hurts really badly!'
Doctor:	'OK. What we can do now is to refer you for an X-ray of your ankle before you are seen by the doctor. Hopefully this will speed up the process and make sure that you are sorted out as quickly as possible.'

Unfortunately, not all patients may respond positively to your efforts to help them. Some may spurn your advice and persist in their demands. If the situation spirals out of control and the patient becomes more angry and violent, then your own personal safety becomes paramount. You should tell the patient that you feel uncomfortable about how things are proceeding and state your intentions that you may terminate the consultation. A firm warning should send a clear message that you are not prepared to continue unless their threats or aggression stops. Your last resort should be to leave the room and call security if you feel the patient has become a danger to yourself or others.

Doctor:	'So, Mr Lewis, I'll get one of the nurses to give you some painkillers right away. There are only two more people in front of you in the queue and hopefully you will be seen shortly.'

Mr Lewis:	'What? You're just gonna give me some paracetamol and disappear off! Typical!'
Doctor:	'I'm really sorry, but I've got patients who are very unwell and need attending to.'
Mr Lewis:	'Look! I am fed up with waiting. Now that I've managed to see a doctor I am not allowing you to leave until I am sorted!'
	PATIENT STANDS UP AGGRESSIVELY SHOUTING
Doctor:	'I am beginning to feel uncomfortable with this situation. I have to warn you that if your behaviour persists then I will have no choice but to leave.'

Summarising back

Having negotiated a solution, it is good practice to summarise back to the patient what has already been agreed. Due to the patient's emotional state, they may not have fully comprehended all that you have said. By offering an opportunity to reflect back to them, any misunderstandings or further concerns can be raised and addressed accordingly.

Doctor:	'So, Mr Lewis, I'd just like to summarise our discussion. I understand that you have injured your ankle and have been waiting for several hours. Unfortunately, because we have been so busy, you've had to wait longer then usual.
	PAUSE
	'We have agreed that I will get one of the nurses to give you some painkillers and in the meantime I will be sending you for an X-ray before you are properly assessed by a doctor. Are you happy with this?'

Closing up

If you have been successful, you will have managed to avert an ugly confrontation between the patient and yourself. By now, they should be a lot more relaxed, and open and content with the agreed plan of action. Any tasks that you have promised to carry out must be fulfilled. Failure to do so will undo all of your hard work and may trigger a more hostile reaction from the patient.

Doctor:	'OK, Mr Lewis. I'll go right away to the X-ray department. The whole process should take about half an hour. If I do get caught up for longer than expected, I'll come out and let you know.'
Mr Lewis:	'You know, Doctor, I don't mind that so much. So long as

I'm informed about what's going on, it'll make me feel a little better.'

Doctor: 'Sure . . . Well, let me crack on with this, and if there is anything else I can do for you, just ask one of the nurses to find me.'

Mr Lewis: 'Thanks for listening, Doctor. I'm sorry for my behaviour earlier.'

Doctor: 'That's fine, Mr Lewis. Let's just concentrate on mending that ankle of yours!'

FIRST CLINICAL SCENARIO

Postponed operation

Dealing with an angry patient is something most doctors will need to tackle at some point in their professional lives. A common scenario would be explaining to a patient that their operation has had to be postponed or cancelled. In such situations it is important that you apologise for the inconvenience and try to offer an acceptable solution.

DOCTOR'S BRIEF

You are the Paediatric Surgical Registrar. You have had an extremely busy day today, and have been stuck in theatre doing your Consultant's operating list. Two patients attended A&E earlier today and both required emergency laparotomies. As a result, surgery has been delayed, and you are unable to fit in the final case due to the CEPOD (emergency surgery) regulations. Your Consultant has given you the task of breaking this news to the parents.

ACTOR'S BRIEF *(if you are the doctor, please do not read)*

You are David Nicols, and you and your wife have come today for your child's herniotomy. You are feeling quite frustrated as you have been waiting all day for your child's surgery. It was supposed to be at midday, and the time is now quarter past five. Your child has been nil by mouth since midnight yesterday, and you are finding it incredibly difficult to control him. You are extremely perturbed by the delay and will display your frustrations if you are told that the operation is postponed or cancelled.

SCENARIO WALK-THROUGH

INTRODUCE YOURSELF TO THE PATIENT'S RELATIVES	*Doctor:*	'Hello, Mr and Mrs Nicols. My name is Mr Khan and I am one of the paediatric surgeons.'
	Mr Nicols:	*'Oh, at last! We've been waiting so long for Jonny's herniotomy. He's been so restless waiting for theatre. He's a handful at the best of times, let alone when he's starving!'*
GIVE EXPLANATION OF CANCELLATION	*Doctor:*	'Mr Nicols, you have been very patient today. Unfortunately, we have had two unexpected emergencies. Although we plan routine surgery well in advance, we do occasionally face unforeseen situations . . .
	PAUSE	
SIGNPOST DIFFICULT NEWS		'Unfortunately, I have some difficult news to tell you.'
	Mr Nicols:	*'What's the matter?'*
GIVE EXPLANATION	*Doctor:*	'Well, due to the extra emergency surgeries we have had to perform today, your son's operation has had to be put back.'
	Mr Nicols:	*'You are joking, aren't you?'*
	Doctor:	'I'm afraid not.'
	Mr Nicols:	*'Do you have any children of your own?'*
	Doctor:	'No.'
ALLOW THE RELATIVES TO VENT THEIR ANGER	*Mr Nicols:*	*'So, you really have no idea! I've been here since eight o'clock this morning with a child who last ate at midnight. Do you realise how difficult that is? No, you probably don't! I know you had two emergencies, but you're telling me now that we can't have the operation today? Why couldn't someone have told us before, instead of making us starve our son for no reason?'*
	Doctor:	'I am sorry that things turned out this way.'
	Mr Nicols:	*'Sorry! SORRY! You have no idea, do you? My son has been running around the ward . . . we have found it so difficult to keep him occupied. He's been crying from hunger and all you can say is sorry?'*
IF RELATIVE'S ANGER IS VALID, TRY TO EMPATHISE	*Doctor:*	'To be perfectly honest, if I was in your position I'd probably be feeling exactly the same as you are right now.'

	Mr Nicols:	'So, the next thing you're probably going to say is that I'm gonna have to wait another few months for the operation.'
ADDRESS RELATIVE'S CONCERNS AND OFFER SOLUTION	Doctor:	'Well . . . I have discussed your case with the Consultant and fortunately he's happy to squeeze you on tomorrow's operation list if you are happy with that.
		'I know that this is no excuse for your experience today but, given the circumstances, I hope that it goes some way in reducing your frustration.'
	Mr Nicols:	'Look, Doctor, I know your work is unpredictable, and today was perhaps a freak occurrence for you guys. I suppose we can wait till tomorrow for the operation. However, it might not have been so bad if someone had kept us informed.'
	Doctor:	'Yes, I'll take that on board. I'll make sure that if there are any further delays, I will personally inform you as soon as possible.'
	Mr Nicols:	'Thank you, Doctor, for explaining this to us.'
SUMMARISE BACK AND CLOSE	Doctor:	'Can I just check that we are in agreement then. Unfortunately your son's operation was cancelled due to two emergency operations. I have rebooked you for first thing tomorrow morning. I apologise for any inconvenience caused and will inform you if there are any further unexpected delays.'
	Mr Nicols:	'OK, Doctor. Thanks for your time. I do appreciate it.'
	Doctor:	'You're welcome. See you soon, Mr Nicols.'

CONSULTATION END

SECOND CLINICAL SCENARIO

Lost referral letter

A common incident that occurs in general practice is when a patient returns frustrated and angry, as they are yet to receive a specialist appointment. What may compound this would be learning that the referral letter had not even been sent by the doctor. In such circumstances, you should apologise unreservedly and offer a frank and honest explanation.

DOCTOR'S BRIEF

You are the GP Registrar at a busy practice. The next patient on your list is Mr Andre Young, a 46-year-old man with a past medical history of chronic back pain. You notice that he has been attending the surgery on a monthly basis during the past year. Browsing through his notes, you see that a referral was made to the Pain Clinic over three months ago. You search for an outpatient clinic letter from the Pain Clinic but cannot find one. You call the Pain Clinic at the hospital and find out that the GP's referral letter was never received. Your task today is to inform the patient that you will have to re-refer them.

ACTOR'S BRIEF *(if you are the doctor, please do not read)*

You are Andre Young, a 46-year-old builder who has been off work for the past 14 months due to back pain which started after an injury at work. You are on a long list of painkillers but these are having less of an effect as each day passes. You were referred to the Pain Clinic three months ago, but haven't yet received an appointment. You feel fed up with waiting for your appointment and would seek private treatment if you could afford it. Your patience is wearing thin, and you have come to the GP today extremely angry about the situation. You realise that mistakes can be made, however, you will lose your temper if you are told that you will need to wait much longer.

SCENARIO WALK-THROUGH

INTRODUCE YOURSELF TO THE PATIENT	*Doctor:*	'Hello, Mr Young. My name is Dr Barrett. How can I help you today?'
	Mr Young:	*'I want to know what the hell is going on with my Pain Clinic appointment! I was referred ages ago and I haven't heard anything!'*
ESTABLISH PATIENT'S CONCERNS	*Doctor:*	'I see. I'm sorry to hear that you have not heard anything. Is there anything in particular that is concerning you about the delay?'
	Mr Young:	*'Are you trying to be funny, Doc? Anything concerning me about the delay? How would you feel if you had to put up with such severe pain that you could not even get out of bed in the morning, and couldn't do anything useful because you are in so much damn pain!'*
ACKNOWLEDGE PATIENT'S CONCERNS	*Doctor:*	'I appreciate your frustration, Mr Young. I'm sorry you have had to put up with such difficulty with your back pain and that you have had to wait so long . . .'
	Mr Young:	*'Enough of that sweet talk, Doc! I've been waiting for over three months and I am fed up!'*
SIGNPOST DIFFICULT NEWS TO FOLLOW	*Doctor:*	'Mr Young, I have made a few phone calls and found out why there has been such a delay. I'm afraid there has been a bit of a mix up.'
	Mr Young:	*'What do you mean, a mix up?'*
	Doctor:	'As you know, you were referred three months ago by one of the other doctors.'
	Mr Young:	*'I know, Doc, get to the point please!'*
	Doctor:	'It appears that unfortunately the original referral letter has been misplaced.'
	Mr Young.	*'Yes, and . . .?'*
	Doctor:	'And because of this it seems that an appointment for you at the Pain Clinic has not been made.'
	Mr Young:	*'You're joking, right?'*
	Doctor:	'I'm afraid not, Mr Young.'
ALLOW THE PATIENT TO VENT THEIR ANGER. DOCTOR SHOULD LISTEN	*Mr Young:*	*'What? It took you three months to find this out! Lost in the post! Lost in the post! I have a right mind to sue you for negligence! What have you people got a degree in? Medicine? But you don't have any*

common sense! I've lost count of the number of times I've come and asked the doctor to find out what the hell has happened to my referral! Do you have any idea how much hell I've gone through with my back? I can't sleep, I can't work, I'm always in pain! It's ruining my life!'

IF PATIENT'S ANGER IS VALID, TRY TO EMPATHISE	

Doctor: 'I am truly sorry, Mr Young, and I fully appreciate why you're angry.'

Mr Young: *'Angry is a massive understatement. I am absolutely livid. If it wasn't for my back, I don't know what I would do . . . I'd, I'd . . .'*

USE OF SILENCE TO AID DEFUSING THE PATIENT'S ANGER	

SILENCE

APPRECIATE PATIENT'S EMOTIONAL RESPONSE	

Doctor: 'Honestly speaking, Mr Young, I would be just as frustrated and angry if it were me. So, I do relate to how you are feeling now.'

Mr Young: *'So, what are you going to do about it then? I am certainly not waiting another three months to be seen.'*

Doctor: 'Once again, I am really sorry for the mix up. What I can do for you now is contact the Consultant directly and explain to them what happened. I am sure they will understand and hopefully they will be able to fit you in as an urgent case. How does that sound?'

Mr Young: *'So, how long would I have to wait? A few days?'*

ADDRESS EXPECTATIONS	

Doctor: 'Well, I can't promise you that. It is more realistic that you'll be seen within a few weeks. You certainly won't be waiting more than that.'

Mr Young: *'Well, if you can sort it out for me, I'd be grateful. How do I know this won't get lost in the system as well?'*

Doctor: 'After I speak to the Consultant, I'll call them back in a couple of days to check they have sent you an appointment.'

Mr Young: *'Well, thanks. I hope it happens this time.'*

Doctor: 'So, can I quickly go over what we have agreed?'

Mr Young: *'OK.'*

SUMMARISE BACK AND CLOSE	*Doctor:*	'Unfortunately, your Pain Clinic appointment was not made due to a lost referral letter. Because of this, you have continued to suffer from your symptoms. To ensure that this does not happen again I will contact the Pain Consultant directly to try to arrange an urgent appointment for you. I'll be contacting you a few days after this to make sure that you have received the appointment. Is that OK?'

Mr Young: *'Thank you, Doctor. I appreciate what you are doing for me.'*

Doctor: 'That's no problem at all. See you soon.'

CONSULTATION END

CHAPTER 5

Explaining medical conditions

Doctors and health professionals are held in high esteem by the general populace due to their ability to piece together patients' complaints in order to arrive at a diagnosis. Such diagnoses may range from a trivial cold to a potentially life-threatening cancer. Although your primary duty as a doctor is to make a provisional diagnosis, it is equally important that you are able to communicate this to the patient and explain its ramifications. It is no longer acceptable practice to merely label the patient with a diagnosis without educating them about it. This task, although it may appear straightforward, often distinguishes between a good clinician and an exceptional one.

Explaining medical conditions requires the practitioner to have a good basic knowledge about the diagnosis, as well as the ability to communicate and simplify complex medical jargon into language that is easily understandable. The clinician will also have to be empathic and be ready to manage a variety of emotional responses that the patient may have.

The skills required are not dissimilar to those already outlined in the previous chapters. Whereas previously, the focus of the consultation was on information gathering *from* the patient, the emphasis in this skill centres around the ability to impart medical information concisely *to* the patient. Although it may be tempting to lecture the patient at length without involving them in the process, a better approach would be to maintain a fluid two-way dialogue where information is exchanged freely. This will result in higher levels of information retention and better patient understanding.

Background knowledge

It goes without saying that before you can explain a medical condition to a patient you should have sufficient knowledge about it. A lot of the patient's trust in your ability will depend on the vast knowledge you hold about medical conditions. If, when you are trying to explain a diagnosis to a patient, you appear to lack confidence and knowledge, the patient's faith in you may be shaken beyond repair. Whilst patients may consider doctors as being 'omniscient', there are literally thousands of medical conditions and you cannot be fully cognisant of them all. Instead you should be fully knowledgeable about common medical conditions that you would be expected to see in your speciality. As a medical student you will be expected to know and explain a number of common generic conditions including:

- Cardiology
  — Hypertension
  — Myocardial infarction
  — Heart failure
- Respiratory medicine
  — Asthma
  — COPD
  — Pneumonia
- Gastroenterology
  — Gastro-oesophageal reflux disease
  — Peptic ulcer disease
  — Inflammatory bowel disease
- Neurology
  — Multiple sclerosis
  — Stroke
  — Epilepsy
- Endocrinology
  — Diabetes
  — Thyroid disease
- Nephrology
  — Acute and chronic renal failure
- Rheumatology
  — Rheumatoid arthritis
  — SLE
- Surgery
  — Bowel cancer

Students often worry about the depth of knowledge they are required to know about each medical condition they encounter. A helpful approach to answer this question would be to ask yourself what information you would like to know if you were the patient.

Learn about the incidence, complications, prognosis and effect on quality of life for the common conditions above. Be prepared, however, to face unexpected questions for which you lack the answers. If you find yourself in such a situation do not speak without knowledge; rather, be honest and state that you do not know but will do your best to find out.

Initiating the consultation

When beginning the consultation, clearly state your name and position. It is better to maintain the formality of the occasion, particularly if you plan to impart difficult news.

Establish rapport by demonstrating an active interest in the patient and their problem. Ask them how they are. As with most consultations, this stage will enable you to determine how the patient is feeling and will guide you in your overall approach. Maintain an open posture and use appropriate body language. Smile. Your aim should be to make the patient feel at ease before they are informed of their diagnosis.

Start off by finding out why the patient is attending today. Do they think that are here for a simple follow-up, a prescription change or for some other reason? This will give the patient an opportunity to mention what they think the purpose of visit is and will help to avoid misunderstandings from the outset. Consider the following example:

Doctor: 'So, now that you have multiple sclerosis, I suppose you know that there is not a great deal we can do for you. Unfortunately, you may end up in a wheelchair. We just have to wait and see . . .'

Patient: 'WHAT? I only came for a repeat prescription . . .!'

Patient's ideas and concerns

Once you have introduced yourself and successfully established rapport, it is essential that you gauge the patient's own understanding of their problems before steamrolling into your explanation. This should make the patient more receptive to the incoming information and more likely to implement the accompanying medical advice.

Ideas: what does the patient already understand?

Patients attend their doctor with preconceived ideas about the symptoms they are suffering. Sometimes they may underestimate the severity of their condition, and other times they may attend with disproportionate anxieties. In most cases patients find it difficult to vocalise their anxieties unless prompted to do so. By asking about their own ideas you give the patient a chance to express these worries in their own words and uncover any inaccuracies in their understanding.

You will often come across patients who already know the basic facts about their disorder and are fully familiar with medical terms and jargon. Such patients may attend with specific demands for a referral or type of treatment. In such cases you should still attempt to establish what the patient already knows before dealing with their request. This will help check that their understanding is correct and allow you modify your explanation accordingly.

Concerns: what is the patient worried about?

Once you have established the patient's own ideas about their problem, it is sensible to elicit any associated concerns that they may have. By doing this the patient may reveal any hidden agendas or concerns that they may be concealing.

In addition to being a vital tool in maintaining rapport with the patient, eliciting their concerns will enable you to focus much of your explanation on that which is relevant to the patient's needs. An example would be explaining the intricacies of epilepsy to a taxi driver whilst making sure you address their foremost concern of how it might affect their vocation.

Remember, concerns can crop up throughout the consultation. When explaining to the patient about their illness, new thoughts and worries may creep into their mind and trouble them. Patients may not volunteer this information directly but may display their anxieties through their body language. It is therefore vital to observe the patient for any signs of unease that may suggest this.

Doctor: 'To prevent your blackouts, Mrs Wood, our team has decided to fit you with a pacemaker. This is a small device that lies just under your skin and delivers pulses of electricity to your heart in order to keep it beating properly and in the right rhythm.'
(Patient's eyebrows rise and she stares at the ground)
Doctor: 'Is there something I have said that is troubling you?'

Explaining the condition

By now you should have obtained some quite detailed and personal information from the patient regarding their condition. Take a step back and consider the possible implications the diagnosis will have on the patient themselves, their family, and their occupation. Comprehending this will allow you to be sensitive and sympathetic in the way you go about delivering any burdensome news.

Summary of the history so far

When explaining the diagnosis to the patient it is always useful to recap their symptoms at presentation. Give one or two sentences that provide a brief overview of the history you have at hand. This will allow the patient an opportunity to correct any inaccuracies and add to the history if need be.

Doctor: 'As you are aware, two weeks ago you experienced an episode

	where your body was shaking uncontrollably, and you were later told you had suffered an epileptic fit. Is that correct?'
Patient:	'Yes, but didn't they tell you that I also bit my tongue and lost control of my bladder?'

Impart the information

You should now proceed to impart the diagnosis using clear language, avoiding jargon, and utilising appropriate pauses. Prioritise the information you give so that the most important points are made first. Pace the delivery of the information you give, checking understanding as you go along. This will allow the patient time to absorb what you have said. It may be helpful to read over the section entitled 'Explaining common conditions' (pp. 96–7) to gain ideas on how to explain these diagnoses.

Doctor:	'Diabetes is a condition that affects the body's ability to control sugar levels. The sugar levels are controlled by a hormone or chemical messenger called insulin.
	PAUSE
	'Unfortunately, your body is not responding to the insulin as well as it used to.
	PAUSE
	'As a result the sugar levels in your blood are consistently high and are causing your symptoms of tiredness, weight loss and passing urine more often.'

Clarity

You should attempt to be clear and unambiguous in your explanation to the patient of their diagnosis. Keep your sentences short and simple and try to avoid complex medical jargon whenever possible. Consider the following example:

Doctor:	'There is a slight possibility that perhaps, although we are not completely sure, that maybe, at some point in the future, you will, as a result of the natural pathological changes which hepatocytes undergo, be left with a liver whose parenchyma has undergone irreversible fibrotic change, and therefore suffer from complications of your excessive intake of alcohol, the consequences of which may or may not be treatable.'
Patient:	'Right. I see. Well, that clears things up!'

Most *doctors* would struggle to understand the above explanation, let alone the patient. A better way to put across the information would be:

Doctor:	'There is a chance that if you continue to drink alcohol excessively your liver will be damaged. *PAUSE* 'The damage may be long lasting and irreversible. *PAUSE* 'It is important to realise that such damage may be untreatable.'

Managing the patient's response and concerns

When informing the patient of a new medical diagnosis, you may be greeted with an array of emotional reactions ranging from complete relief to outbursts of anger. Conditions that are life threatening or life changing will often generate similar emotions as those when breaking bad news to a patient. In such cases you should offer the patient ample time to collect their thoughts and emotions before going on to divulge further information. It may be useful to ask whether they wish to have a friend or family member present before proceeding. Much of this has already been discussed and can be reviewed in Chapter 2 on breaking bad news.

New concerns

Having been told of their diagnosis, the patient may have new thoughts and worries rushing through their head. They may be thinking about how long they have to live, the impact on their day-to-day life and whether or not they can return to full-time employment. Never attempt to brush aside these concerns; rather, you should address them at the earliest opportunity.

Patient:	'So, I am diabetic! That's the end of my career then!'
Doctor:	'Why do you think that is?'
Patient:	'Didn't I tell you? I have been driving an articulated lorry for the last 15 years and now I am going to lose my licence because of my diabetes!'
Doctor:	'Well, as far as I understand from the DVLA regulations, the type of diabetes that you have been diagnosed with should not cause an automatic ban. Your diabetes should respond well with diet and medication therapy and if monitored well you may not need to take insulin injections.'

Check understanding

It may appear that the patient has fully understood everything you have said. However, bear in mind that most patients will not volunteer their ignorance for fear of embarrassment. Hence, it would be prudent for you to check their understanding at regular intervals throughout the consultation.

Doctor: 'We have discussed a lot of things today in a very short space of time. Is there anything that I could have said more clearly or that you would like me to go over?'

Patient: 'Yes, Doctor. Actually, there was something. The bit about . . .'

By checking the patient's understanding, you might occasionally uncover a misconception that they hold. Elicit these and address them as appropriate.

Doctor: 'I appreciate that you are worried about the complications of having another angiogram, and the thought of having a mesh in your blood vessel concerns you. However, I would like to point out that your chances of being pain-free are very good if the procedure is successful.'

Patient: 'But I heard you could treat my problem with a bypass operation? I'm not too keen on these modern keyhole methods, Doctor.'

Doctor: 'I appreciate your concerns. As I mentioned earlier, the advantages of angioplasty and stent insertion over traditional bypass surgery are immense. You will not need a general anaesthetic, your recovery time will be extremely quick so you can return to normal life sooner, and the rate of complications is much lower.'

Agree on a course of action

Once the patient has been informed of their diagnosis, they will naturally go on to enquire what can be done about it. Can it be cured? Will they die a premature death? Is it contagious or hereditary? Your job as the physician would be to try, to the best of your ability, to answer such questions and arrive at a shared course of action, i.e. management plan.

The plan may be something as simple as agreeing to a follow-up appointment with the patient to discuss things further. However, more commonly, you would be required to give a very brief overview of the treatment options available. This may give the patient food for thought prior to your next encounter with them.

Patient: 'Now I have been diagnosed with diabetes, what can I do about it?'

Doctor: 'We have a number of treatment options available that can help control your diabetes. The first and most important way would be to reduce your sugar intake and your weight. In most cases diet alone is enough to keep the sugar level in check.'

Patient: 'And what if that does not work, Doc?'

Doctor: 'In that case, we could start you on some tablets that will help reduce your sugar levels. We have a number of different medications which can do this. If these are unsuccessful, the final step would be to consider insulin injections, but only as a last resort.'

Patient: 'Alright, Doc. I think that there is a lot for me to think about. Is it OK if I have some time to think things over and get back to you?'

You may find on occasions that the patient's line of questioning about their disorder is beyond your depth of knowledge. In such situations it is much better for you to admit your limitations and offer the patient a specialist referral if so desired.

Summarising back

Before concluding the consultation with the patient, it is good practice to summarise back a brief synopsis of what has been discussed. This will not only reinforce the information that you have given but also allow the patient the opportunity to voice any new concerns or questions.

Doctor: 'So, Mr Smith, before we finish I would just like to go over what has been mentioned today and what the plan is. If there is something you don't quite understand or are unsure about, please do stop me.

PAUSE

'Your tests have shown that you suffer from diabetes. We agreed that initially the best course of treatment would be to focus on your diet and avoid sugary foods like cakes, biscuits and fizzy drinks. We also mentioned that you should reduce your fatty food intake by avoiding fast foods.

PAUSE

'Hopefully these measures will bring your sugar levels under control and we will recheck them in six to eight weeks' time when I will be seeing you again.'

Closing up

You are now close to ending your consultation with the patient. Your patient has been labelled with a new diagnosis which perhaps they do not fully understand. It is likely that the patient is overwhelmed with confused thoughts and emotions, which have affected their ability to digest everything you have said. Hence, they may need time to mull things over, discuss with friends and family, or perhaps do some personal research before coming back to see you again. Offer the patient a suitable follow-up appointment which will give them an opportunity to discuss with you any new issues that have arisen. Give the patient an information leaflet that summarises the salient points of the consultation.

You may wish to advise the patient about relevant support groups that they can contact for further information about their diagnosis. Many such groups have good resource materials and contain a wealth of knowledge and experience particularly aimed at newly diagnosed patients.

Doctor: 'Before we end today, I would like to give you a leaflet that talks about your diagnosis in a little more detail. It also has information about patient groups and websites that you may wish to contact.'

Patient: 'Thanks, Doctor, I'll have a read on the way home.'

Doctor: 'Right then, I hope everything goes well for you. I'll hopefully see you in four weeks' time.'

Patient: 'Thanks again. See you next time.'

EXPLAINING COMMON CONDITIONS

When explaining a diagnosis to a patient, it is important to make your explanation as understandable as possible. In order to do this you should try to avoid medical jargon wherever possible and try to simplify complex concepts into language that the patient will understand. Below are examples of ways one can explain common conditions to a patient.

Hypertension

'The heart is a pump that pushes blood around your body. The pressure that forces blood around is known as the blood pressure. The pressure at which blood flows away from your heart (when it contracts) is known as the systolic pressure, whilst the pressure when the heart is at rest is known as the diastolic pressure.

'Blood pressure is normally expressed as a fraction with the upper number representing the systolic pressure and lower number being the diastolic pressure. High blood pressure is when your blood pressure is greater than 140 over 80 (140/80).

'There is no single cause of high blood pressure; rather, a number of factors play a role in causing it. For example, having too much salt in your diet, being obese and not doing enough physical exercise, all contribute to raised blood pressure. Adjusting these factors will help control it.'

Hypercholesterolaemia

'Cholesterol is the name of a fatty substance found in your blood. It is made in the body after breaking down the saturated fats from your diet. Broadly speaking, there are two types of cholesterol, low density (LDL) and high density (HDL). Low density or LDL cholesterol carries the fat into cells of the body. High density or HDL cholesterol, removes any excess cholesterol from the body by breaking it down in the liver.

'In principle, HDL cholesterol is good while LDL cholesterol is bad. Too much LDL cholesterol in the blood can cause a build up in your blood vessels and slowly over time cause a blockage. A blockage in the vessels of the brain is known as a stroke, whilst a blockage in the vessels of the heart is known as a heart attack.

'A poor diet high in saturated fats, and a lack of exercise, will put you at risk of developing high cholesterol.'

Gastro-oesophageal reflux disease (GORD)

'Your stomach produces acid which helps it break down food. If some of this acid leaks back into your food pipe, this is known as acid reflux. When this happens you may feel heartburn, which is a burning feeling that starts from your stomach and moves up to your throat. This may also cause an unpleasant taste in the back of your mouth.

'Smoking, alcohol and caffeine are known to make reflux worse. They do this by relaxing the muscle at the junction between your food pipe and your stomach, allowing acid to reflux. Being overweight or pregnant can increase the pressure on your stomach and also produce the same symptoms. Certain foods, such as spices, chilli and fried food, can affect the way the stomach works and increase its acid content, thereby causing discomfort.'

Asthma

'Asthma is a condition that affects your lungs. Your lungs are made up of lots of small tubes that allow air, and in particular oxygen, to pass freely. In asthma, certain triggers, also known as allergens, may irritate these airways and cause them to become narrow. As a result air may become trapped inside your lungs making you feel short of breath. The narrowed airways also restrict the flow of air through them making your chest feel tight, as well as producing a sound known as a wheeze.

'Common allergens include dust mites, pollen, cigarette smoke and infections.'

FIRST CLINICAL SCENARIO

Myocardial infarction

Patients come through A&E unwell and sometimes in a critical state. They may have a basic understanding as to what is going on but want to seek reassurance that nothing serious is amiss. Hence, when breaking the news of the diagnosis to the patient you should be sensitive and anticipate possible heightened emotional responses.

DOCTOR'S BRIEF

You are the Foundation Year House Officer in Cardiology. Mr Dave Stevenson is a 58-year-old publican who presented to casualty yesterday with chest pain. He is a smoker and suffers from hypertension and hyperlipidaemia. His ECG was normal but his cardiac enzymes were elevated confirming a non-ST-elevation myocardial infarction. He seems to be doing extremely well and has not suffered any complications. Your Consultant expects he will recover well. He has been told that he has had a heart attack, but has little idea about what this diagnosis means and what impact it will have on his life. Give accurate information regarding the diagnosis, the effect on his lifestyle and your plan for continuing management. You do not need to give any explanation regarding the inpatient investigations.

ACTOR'S BRIEF *(if you are the doctor, please do not read)*

You are Dave Stevenson, a 58-year-old publican. You were told yesterday whilst you were being admitted that you had suffered a heart attack and that you had had a 'lucky escape'.

You know extremely little about what a heart attack is and have no idea about how it will affect your life. You want to know more about it and what the plan is regarding your treatment. You are concerned about your future health and what precautions you need to take once you have gone home. You are happy to follow any advice you are given and would be willing to attend any follow-up appointments.

SCENARIO WALK-THROUGH

INTRODUCE YOURSELF TO THE PATIENT AND ESTABLISH RAPPORT	*Doctor:*	'Hello, Mr Stevenson. I'm Dr Jones. How are you today?'
	Mr S:	*'Not bad, Doctor. I feel a bit better today.'*
	Doctor:	'I'm pleased to hear that. I was hoping to talk to you about what has happened to you recently.'
	Mr S:	*'Yes, that would be good.'*
ESTABLISH PATIENT'S IDEAS	*Doctor:*	'I was wondering if you could tell me what led you to come into hospital?'
	Mr S:	*'Well, to be honest, Doctor, all I know is that one moment I was having chest pain, and the next moment I'd been rushed to hospital.'*
ESTABLISH PATIENT'S CONCERNS	*Doctor:*	'OK. Is there anything in particular that you are worried about?'
	Mr S:	*'Well, I'm worried about what is going to happen to me. Am I alright? Will this affect my job or my life?'*
	Doctor:	'I appreciate your concerns. I'm sure it is quite worrying being in hospital under these circumstances.
	PAUSE	
SHOW EMPATHY AND ESTABLISH PATIENT'S EXPECTATIONS		'I would like to go through a few things regarding your admission and hopefully deal with some of your concerns. Is there anything in particular you would like me to discuss with you today?'
DEMONSTRATE ACTIVE LISTENING (EYE CONTACT, OPEN BODY POSTURE)	*Mr S:*	*'Well, nothing specific Doctor. I just want to know what's happening to me!'*
SUMMARY OF HISTORY SO FAR	*Doctor:*	'Well, as you know, yesterday you experienced an episode of chest pain. You were brought into hospital by an ambulance and given some emergency treatment to ease the pain.
SPACE INFORMATION APPROPRIATELY		'We performed a few tests, and those tests confirmed that you had suffered from a heart attack.'
	Mr S:	*'I am sorry, Doctor, for sounding stupid but can you tell me exactly what that means?'*
	Doctor:	'OK, that's not a problem. Your heart is essentially a pump which pushes blood around the body so that your organs and tissues can receive oxygen and food.

PAUSE

GIVE INFORMATION
IN BITE-SIZE
PORTIONS

'The heart itself is a muscle and requires its own oxygen and nutrients to keep it working properly. These travel in the blood to the heart by specific vessels.

PAUSE

'Over time, these vessels can become narrowed because of cholesterol. Eventually, the vessel can become so narrowed – or even block completely – that the heart muscle is starved of oxygen.

PAUSE

'Due to the lack of oxygen, this area of heart muscle can be permanently damaged and die. When this happens your body produces an intense pain similar to what you experienced yesterday.'

Mr S: *'What can I do to stop it happening again?'*

Doctor: 'There are a few things which put a person at increased risk of having a heart attack. These include smoking, as in your case, high blood pressure, high cholesterol, diabetes and having a family history of heart disease.

'By controlling these risk factors we should be able to reduce the chances of this happening again. Our aim will be to reduce your blood pressure and cholesterol, encourage you to do things such as lose weight, eat a healthy diet and quit smoking.

'Are you happy with what we have discussed so far?'

CHECK PATIENT'S
UNDERSTANDING OF
INFORMATION GIVEN

Mr S: *'Yes, Doctor. What about my heart? Will it get better?'*

Doctor: 'Unfortunately, the areas which have been damaged will not get better but rather heal as scar tissue. As long as the damage is not too severe the heart should function close to normal.'

Mr S: *'So, I guess I'm going to have to take it easy from now on. Is there anything I need to do or avoid?'*

Doctor: 'You will need to be careful for the first few days after you get home, during which time you should avoid heavy lifting and walking long distances.

Gradually, you should build up your level of exercise as much as you can tolerate.

'Cold weather can sometimes make chest pain come on sooner, so make sure you wrap up warm when outside.

'In terms of driving, it is important you let your insurance company know. As long as you recover normally, you can resume driving after four weeks. If you get chest pains when driving, you should stop until your symptoms are under control.

'In general, as long as you recover well, sexual activity can resume after four weeks.'

Mr S: *'So, what's going to happen to me now?'*

AGREE ON A PLAN

Doctor: 'Well, we have started you on two medications to thin your blood. This will help prevent blockages developing in your heart vessels again. We have also increased the dosage of your blood pressure medications and your cholesterol tablets as studies have shown that they are beneficial in people who have had heart attacks.

'Finally, you have been given a pink spray to use under the tongue if you ever feel a similar type of pain to what you experienced when you first came in.

PAUSE

CHECK PATIENT'S UNDERSTANDING

'We have gone through quite a lot of information today. Is there anything that you wish me to go over?'

Mr S: *'No. What you have said makes a lot of sense. What will happen next?'*

Doctor: 'We will continue to monitor your progress. It is likely that as you recover you will undergo further tests to investigate the condition of your heart and the extent of the narrowing of the heart vessels. You will be told more about these tests nearer the time.

OFFER FOLLOW-UP

'We will also refer you to the cardiac rehabilitation service who will give you detailed information and advice as to your specific needs. They will continue to see you after you have been discharged home from the ward. Is that OK?'

	Mr S:	*'Yes, Doctor.'*
CHECK PATIENT'S UNDERSTANDING AND ENCOURAGE QUESTIONS	*Doctor:*	'Is there anything that you want to clarify?'
	Mr S:	*'No, Doctor, you have made yourself very clear.'*
	Doctor:	'Do you have any more questions?'
	Mr S:	*'No, not at the moment.'*
SUMMARISE BACK AND CHECK PATIENT'S UNDERSTANDING AGAIN	*Doctor:*	'If it is OK then, I'll just briefly go over what we've discussed. (Patient nods in agreement)
		'Yesterday, you came into hospital with chest pain and after a few tests we found that you had suffered a heart attack.
		'We started you on a number of medications to protect your heart from any further damage and increased your tablets to reduce the risk of another heart attack.
		'Whilst you are on the ward we will continue to monitor you and only discharge you once you are medically fit.
		'We hope to see you again in our clinics to carry out some more tests. Is there anything else which you wanted to add or ask?'
	Mr S:	*'Thanks, Doctor. You have been very helpful.'*
CONCLUDE AND CLOSE	*Doctor:*	'Thank you for your time, Mr Stevenson. I'll see you again soon.'

CONSULTATION END

SECOND CLINICAL SCENARIO

Systemic lupus erythematosus (SLE)

In the outpatient setting, the patient is likely to be stable and clinically well. Many patients would have been given some idea as to what their diagnosis is by their GP. Some patients may have done extensive research prior to their appointment and come armed with a barrage of questions. Some, on the other hand, may remain blissfully unaware of their diagnosis. However well informed the patient is, it is important to check their understanding. Although certain chronic conditions may not be immediately life threatening to the patient, they may nevertheless be the cause of a great deal of angst and worry.

DOCTOR'S BRIEF

You are the Foundation Year House Officer in Rheumatology. Mrs Joanna Lawrence is a 33-year-old woman of African–Caribbean origin who has been complaining of joint pains, muscle aches and tiredness for the past few months. More recently she has also noticed a rash appearing on her cheeks. The GP has performed blood tests which were positive for anti-nuclear antigen and anti-double stranded DNA antibodies. The GP has warned the patient that she may be suffering from lupus and has referred her to your Consultant's clinic for further information.

ACTOR'S BRIEF *(if you are the doctor, please do not read)*

You are Joanna Lawrence, a 33-year-old woman of African–Caribbean origin. You have come to the Rheumatology clinic today after receiving a letter from the hospital.

You are expecting to find out more about the results of the blood tests which your GP has carried out. You have absolutely no idea about what lupus is despite being told by your GP that you are suffering from this. You are anxious to learn more from the specialist about the illness and the treatment options.

SCENARIO WALK-THROUGH

<table>
<tr>
<td>

INTRODUCE YOURSELF
TO THE PATIENT AND
ESTABLISH RAPPORT
</td>
<td>

Doctor:
</td>
<td>

'Hello, Mrs Lawrence. I'm Dr Edwards. How are you today?'
</td>
</tr>
</table>

INTRODUCE YOURSELF TO THE PATIENT AND ESTABLISH RAPPORT

Doctor: 'Hello, Mrs Lawrence. I'm Dr Edwards. How are you today?'

Mrs L: *'I'm fine, thank you.'*

ESTABLISH PATIENT'S IDEAS

Doctor: 'I understand that your GP referred you for the results of blood tests you have had. Is that correct? Can you tell me what you have been told so far?'

Mrs L: *'My GP told me that I might have something called lupus and that I should speak to you to find out more about it.'*

Doctor: 'That's quite right. I'm here to explain your diagnosis and answer any questions you may have. Do you know anything about lupus already?'

Mrs L: *'Not much actually. All I know is that it's causing this rash on my face and causing my arm pains.'*

ESTABLISH PATIENT'S CONCERNS

DEMONSTRATE ACTIVE LISTENING (EYE CONTACT, OPEN BODY POSTURE)

Doctor: 'I see. Is there anything in particular that concerns or worries you about lupus?'

Mrs L: *'Well, it's come as a bit of a shock, to be honest. I mean, can it be treated? I am worried about what else will happen to me apart from this rash and the pains.'*

Doctor: 'Today, I would like to go through a few things about your diagnosis and deal with any concerns that you may have.'

Mrs L: *'Yes, that's fine.'*

SUMMARY OF HISTORY SO FAR

Doctor: 'From your GP's letter I understand that for the past few months you have felt more tired than usual and that occasionally your joints have hurt. Recently, you visited your GP after a rash developed on your face and you had several blood tests performed.

PAUSE

SPACE INFORMATION APPROPRIATELY

'From the history and the blood test results it appears that you are suffering with a condition called systemic lupus erythematosus, or lupus for short.'

Mrs L: *'Hmm, I see.'*

Doctor: 'Lupus is an autoimmune disorder. This mean that your immune system, which normally fights foreign infections, incorrectly turns on itself and begins to attack the body causing inflammation and swelling.

PAUSE

'In the case of lupus, this inflammation can cause a wide variety of symptoms including a rash, muscle aching and joint swelling.'

Mrs L: 'Yes, but what causes it?'

Doctor: 'Unfortunately, we do not yet have the answer for that. There are various theories but nothing has so far been proven. We have found that it mainly occurs in young people and is more commonly seen in African–Caribbean and Asian women.'

Mrs L: 'So, can you treat it?'

Doctor: 'Although no cure has been found we are able to manage many of the symptoms. Treatment aims to prevent flare-ups and to reduce the amount of inflammation which is present.

'Your treatment will depend on the severity of your illness. The vast majority of patients with lupus suffer from a mild form requiring no treatment at all. If, however, you are symptomatic with aches and stiffness of the joints, you may be prescribed some analgesia to reduce this.

'If your symptoms become more intense and severe we might have to treat you with some steroid tablets to reduce the inflammation until the symptoms are under control, and then we will aim to lower the dose or stop it completely.

PAUSE

'In the unlikely event that your lupus does not respond to this treatment, there are a number of other drugs that we can consider at a later stage.'

Mrs L: 'Will it get worse?'

Doctor: 'In most people, there are long periods where the illness is mild and symptoms are few. This period is known as remission.

PAUSE

'When a flare-up occurs, and symptoms become worse, it is called a relapse. It is difficult to predict when relapses will occur and how severe they will be. Be sure to seek medical advice when you feel your symptoms are worsening.

PAUSE

CHECK PATIENT'S UNDERSTANDING

'I know I have given you a lot of information in a very short time. I was wondering if there's anything that I have said that you wish me to clarify?'

Mrs L: *'No, Doctor. You have been quite clear . . . So, what now?'*

AGREE ON A PLAN

Doctor: 'The Consultant has prescribed you some medications which will help control your symptoms. You will need to have regular blood tests in the future, which will give us information about the severity of the disease. You will be seen again by the Consultant in a few weeks' time.

(Patient appears worried and breaks into tears)

DEMONSTRATE UNDERSTANDING AND SHOW EMPATHY

Doctor: 'I understand it can be quite overwhelming to be informed of a new diagnosis. I am sure it can be quite difficult to come to terms with this. Is there anything I could do to help?' *(Doctor offers a box of tissues)*

Mrs L: *'No, Doctor. You have been terrific.'*

Doctor: 'It may be an idea to talk to your family and friends about it or consider getting in touch with patient groups who will be able to offer you a wealth of experience. Does that sound OK?'

Mrs L: *'That sounds fine. Thank you for your advice.'*

OFFERS SPECIALIST NURSE FOLLOW-UP

Doctor: 'I think it may be a good idea if you see Sue, our specialist lupus nurse. She can see you in a couple of days. She is very knowledgeable about lupus and also very approachable. If you have any questions I am sure she will be happy to discuss them with you.'

Mrs L: *'Thank you. I think that is a very good idea.'*

SUMMARISE BACK AND CHECK PATIENT'S UNDERSTANDING AGAIN

Doctor: 'If it is OK then, I'll just briefly go over what we've discussed so far.

'You had blood tests which showed that you suffer from lupus. We discussed this today and I explained

that the majority of people suffer from a mild
form that requires no treatment. If, however, your
symptoms worsen we can consider painkillers or even
steroid tablets to get them under control.

PAUSE

'We hope to see you in a few weeks' time and I will
also be putting you in touch with Sue, our specialist
lupus nurse.

OFFERS PATIENT
INFORMATION
LEAFLET

'Here is a short information leaflet containing the key
facts about lupus. It may be an idea to read over this
before you see Sue.

'Is there anything else which you wanted to add or
ask?'

Mrs L: 'No thanks, Doctor.'

CONCLUDE AND CLOSE

Doctor: 'Thank you for your time, Mrs Lawrence.'

CONSULTATION END

CHAPTER 6

Explaining medical procedures

Patients routinely undergo various medical investigations and procedures on a daily basis. These may be simple procedures, such as a blood test or an ECG, or more complex ones, such as an ERPC (Endoscopic Retrograde Cholangio-Pancreatography). Medical technology has advanced immensely in the past two decades and there are now numerous tests and investigations available for the doctor's use. Although these tests may be essential for the physician to arrive at a diagnosis, some are quite invasive and carry the risk of serious complications. As a result, the patient's agreement must be sought explicitly before proceeding.

When explaining a procedure to the patient, it is essential that you keep things simple and avoid any complex medical terminologies. Patients are often anxious and apprehensive about undergoing a procedure and the use of complicated jargon will only compound this. Good communication and a simple explanation will help allay any fears and will result in a more contented patient.

The General Medical Council (GMC) encourages those who perform the procedure to personally gain consent from the patient. This is because they have greater expertise and understanding of what it entails and ultimately would be held responsible if things were to go wrong. Unfortunately, due to the multiple commitments of senior staff members, they are not always available to do this. More often than not, a junior doctor is burdened with this duty.

In order to be competent in this task, it is essential that you prepare yourself with background knowledge about the procedure, side effects and possible complications that may result. Failure to do so may lead you to consent patients inadequately, leaving you open to liability if things were to go wrong.

Informed consent
Consenting had often involved a junior doctor simply handing over a form to the patient to sign a few moments before they were whisked away to

theatre – blissfully unaware of what to expect. This is no longer acceptable practice. The GMC advises that for informed consent to have taken place, three requirements have to be fulfilled. The first of these consists of the patient being given an adequate explanation of the procedure or investigation being offered. This explanation should cover key points that are relevant to the procedure at hand and should include a description of what will take place, possible side effects and complications.

The second requirement is that the patient must offer their consent voluntarily without coercion. Although clinicians would like to believe that they always act in the best interests of the patient, the patient's own circumstances, wants and desires should take precedence. It is important to remember that the patient is the one who has to undergo the procedure and bear the brunt of any ensuing complications.

The last requirement is that the patient must have the mental capacity to give informed consent. They will need the capability to understand and retain the information you give them as well as communicate their decision back to you. Although the vast majority of patients will have no problems with this, you should be wary of a small minority of people who do lack capacity and will require specialist input.

Types of consent

In some situations, consent may be *implied* by the patient. This may take the form of a patient removing their shirt for an examination or rolling up their sleeve for routine blood testing. In such cases, implied consent should be sufficient for you to perform the task without recourse to documentation. On the other hand, for intimate or complex procedures where there is significant risk of harm, it is important to gain *explicit* written consent from the patient. This is to ensure that if things were to go wrong, there is written evidence that the patient had been made fully aware of the potential risks and subsequent sequelae.

Background knowledge

When explaining a medical procedure to a patient to gain consent, it is vital that the physician doing so has ample knowledge about it. An inaccurate description may leave the patient anxious and confused, causing them to decline the procedure from the outset. A similar outcome may also occur if your explanation is too complex or technical. Therefore, a balanced approach must be sought in order to attain informed consent.

Students often question the need to get 'sign-ups' for viewing common medical procedures in their early clinical years. Whilst they may be tedious exercises at the time, they help you gain first-hand knowledge of the processes from start to finish and a true understanding of what they entail – such opportunities are few and far between after you have qualified as a doctor.

Whilst viewing the procedure will form a good foundation to your knowledge, you should supplement this with additional reading. There are numerous sources of quality information, including patient information leaflets, textbooks and web-based resources such as online videos. Patient information leaflets are a particularly good resource for revision as they are often well structured, with good diagrams and clear, thoughtful, jargon-free explanations – ideal for OSCE examinations.

Common procedures

Whilst it may be unreasonable to expect the average doctor to know about the risks and benefits of *all* procedures, there are a number of common ones that you will be expected to know, both for exams as well as when you become a junior doctor. These include:

- Imaging – CT scanning, MRI scanning, nuclear imaging (V/Q scan)
- Endoscopic procedures – oesophago-gastro-duodenoscopy (OGD), colonoscopy, bronchoscopy
- Contrast studies – barium swallow, barium meal, barium follow-through
- Anaesthetics – induction of general anaesthesia, epidural, spinal anaesthesia, pain management
- Surgery procedures – laparoscopic cholecystectomy, transurethral resection of prostate (TURP), tonsillectomy, hemicolectomy, joint replacement.

Avoiding jargon

When explaining medical procedures to patients, you should try your utmost to avoid using medical terms. It is useful, therefore, to have in your vocabulary a list of simple terms that you can use instead. Consider the following examples:

- Scope   *'Camera'*
- Endoscopy   *'Camera test'*
- Biopsy   *'Sample of tissue', or 'sample from the lining of . . .'*
- Analgesia   *'Painkillers'*
- Sedation   *'Something to make you feel sleepy'*
- Laparoscopy   *'Keyhole surgery'*
- Venflon   *'Small plastic tube'*
- Suture   *'Stitch'*
- Cytology   *'Cell examination'*
- Histology   *'Sample examined under a microscope'*

- Malignancy   *'Cancer' or 'tumour'*
- Metastasis   *'Spread of cancer to other sites'*
- Haemorrhage   *'Bleed'*
- Myocardial infarction   *'Heart attack'*
- Hypertension   *'Blood pressure'*

Initiating the consultation

Often the patient will know very little about the procedure they are about to undergo. They may have been misinformed by an unreliable online source or by misguided friends or family. As a result, they may be feeling apprehensive and anxious before they enter the consultation. It is, therefore, paramount that the introductory stages of the interview are well handled so that the patient feels at ease and willing to discuss their fears and concerns with you.

Doctor: 'Hello, Mr Evans. My name is Dr White. How are you today?'

Mr Evans: 'Not too bad, Doctor, you know, plodding along as usual!'

Doctor: 'That's good! Do you know why I have asked you to attend today?'

Mr Evans: 'Erm . . . not really, Doctor. To be quite honest, I thought I was having a medical before the procedure, you know, like a quick MOT!'

Doctor: 'Well, that's partly true, but the main purpose of today is just to spend a little more time talking about this operation you're going to have.'

Patient's ideas and concerns

Most patients have some understanding about their procedure but may have incorrect ideas and notions of what to expect. By addressing these head-on you are more likely to persuade the patient to consent to the procedure and relieve any underlying anxieties.

Doctor: 'Your GP has requested us to perform an MRI scan of your head. Before I begin, can you tell me what you already know about an MRI scan?'

Patient: 'I don't know much about them, Doctor. I read off the internet that they will put me in some big machine and zap my head with X-rays.'

Doctor: 'Hmm . . . Do you have any worries about having the MRI then?'

Patient: 'Well . . . actually yes. I read that X-rays can cause cancer. Won't all of these X-rays give me brain cancer, Doc?'

Doctor:	'Well, today I hope that I can explain a little bit more about what an MRI scan is and put you at ease regarding your worries.'

Sometimes, it can be difficult to elicit the patient's concerns, perhaps due to embarrassment about the nature of the procedure, e.g. colonoscopy. In such situations, establishing sound rapport and empathising with the patient should help to gain their trust. Consider the example below:

Doctor:	'Miss Brown, you seem to be a little concerned about your colonoscopy? Would you like to talk about it?'
Miss Brown:	'Not really, Doctor. It's kind of personal.' *PAUSE*
Doctor:	'I would just like to say that everything we discuss today is held in the strictest confidence. It would be helpful to know your concerns about the test as perhaps by understanding these issues, I can try to address them better.'
Miss Brown:	'Well, I've had one of these before . . . and . . . it kind of reminded me . . . of a difficult encounter I had a few years ago . . . when my ex-boyfriend forced himself on me . . .' *(Starts crying)* *(Doctor hands her a tissue and gives her a glass of water)*

Explaining the procedure

When explaining the procedure to the patient you should always start by informing them what procedure they are about to have and what it involves. State in simple words the nature of the investigation and the reason why it is being done, for example:

Doctor:	'The test you will be having is known as an OGD endoscopy. The endoscope is a long thin flexible tube with a camera at one end. It allows the doctor to look closely at the lining of the food pipe, stomach and the first part of the intestine.'

Describing the journey

Studies have shown that individuals retain information better when it is presented in a logical and sequential manner. When attempting to explain a procedure to a patient, it is useful to divide it into a chronology of events encompassing pre-op, during and post-op. A simple approach would be to describe the procedure from the patient's point of view as if it were a journey. You should explain who they may meet along that journey, what they should expect and what may be done to them. Adopting this method will not only simplify your explanation, but also ensure that you do not miss out any crucial bits of information.

Pre-op

Pre-op is the period before the procedure. This is the time when the patient waits patiently for their investigation and is likely to be at their most vulnerable. Hence, if faced with anything unexpected during this time, the patient may become anxious and want to cancel or reschedule the procedure. Therefore, it is important that you adequately brief the patient of what to expect.

Explain to the patient the time they should arrive and warn them of the need to change into hospital attire. A number of procedures require the patient to be medically prepped, i.e. by being nil by mouth overnight or being given bowel-cleansing solutions. These should be thoroughly explained to the patient as poor preparation may lead to inadequate views, requiring the procedure to be repeated unnecessarily.

Be careful to avoid overloading the patient with too much information. It may be tempting to rush through your explanation, as demonstrated in the following example:

Doctor: 'It is really quite straightforward. On the morning of the procedure you will be greeted by the ward sister and she will escort you to your bed. Then one of the doctors will come and clerk you in. After that they will insert a cannula into your vein and then give you some fluids. When the time of the operation comes you will be taken to the induction room, where you will meet the anaesthetist. He will give you some pre-med, and then once that takes effect he will give you an induction agent which will put you to sleep. Is that clear?'

It would be better for you to present the above information using bite-sized amounts that are well spaced out.

Doctor: 'Before the procedure, you will be taken to the anaesthetic room and that is where you will meet the anaesthetist who will put you to sleep during the procedure. He will be with you throughout the operation, monitoring various things, from your heart rate to your breathing, to make sure everything is OK.'

Mr Evans: 'That's good to know!'

Doctor: 'He will start off by popping a small plastic tube into a vein so that he can give you medicine quickly. Initially, he might give you some medicine that will relax you a little. *PAUSE*

'After that you will be given an oxygen mask to breathe through before being given the anaesthetic. Hopefully within a few seconds you'll be fast asleep and will not feel a thing.'

During the procedure

This part of the explanation is probably the most important and relevant to the patient in order for you to gain informed consent. It should include a thorough discussion of what will be done and possible side effects that may be experienced. Patients often worry about pain and discomfort during the procedure and this should be addressed honestly and frankly.

Doctor: 'You will be brought in from the pre-op room to the endoscopic suite. The doctor will check once more that you are happy to proceed and then insert a mouth guard to keep your mouth open. The thin endoscope will be passed painlessly into your stomach and photos will be taken. *PAUSE*

'During the procedure, air may be puffed into your stomach to allow a clearer view. The doctor may take a small sample of tissue or a biopsy from inside using tiny forceps. *PAUSE*

'This should not cause any discomfort. The whole procedure may last up to half an hour.'

Recovery phase

To complete the journey, inform the patient about the post-procedural phase and what they would expect to see and experience. Patients often wake up after a procedure feeling disorientated and confused. Simply warning them about this may help ease their anxiety when they pass through this phase. If relevant, advise the patient the need to bring a friend or family member to take them home after the procedure.

Doctor: 'When the endoscopy is finished, you will be taken into a recovery room. You will normally remain there for about an hour to allow time for the sedative to wear off. You may feel a little sick, or bloated and complain of a sore throat. These symptoms are quite normal and usually wear off after a few days.

PAUSE

'After the procedure you will probably still feel tired for the rest of the day and you should bring someone with you to take you home.'

Complications

Every medical procedure has risks and complications. These can range from minor problems to life-threatening emergencies. When explaining the procedure to the patient you should always ensure that you spend time discussing both intra- and post-procedural complications with them. Whilst mentioning a list of complications may alarm the patient, you should always put this into perspective by stating their incidence and rates of occurrence.

Doctor: 'With any medical procedure there are risks and complications that can occur, but thankfully these are rare. Some of these include infection, bleeding and even puncturing of the food pipe. It is important to note, however, that the chances of any of these happening are extremely low (i.e. less than one in a thousand per procedure). However, our staff are well prepared and trained to deal with these complications should any of them occur. Are you happy to go ahead?'

Check understanding

It is always good to check that the patient has understood what you have said before continuing. This process is particularly important when consenting the patient before any procedure.

Elicit any further concerns

You have now explained to the patient about the procedure and given them lots of information, which may take some time to digest. In addition, the patient may also have developed new concerns about the procedure which are yet to be elicited. Attempt to address these by simply asking the patient whether or not they are still happy to proceed and if they have any new concerns.

If the patient is happy to go ahead, it may be an appropriate time to document the discussion in the notes and complete a consent form with them. If written consent is sought, stress to the patient that they can still change their mind at any stage before the procedure.

Follow-up

Results of investigations or procedures are rarely available immediately after the procedure has been completed. More often than not, a skilled technician or specialist is required to interpret the results before providing a detailed report. Warn the patient that it may take a few weeks for this process to be completed. Offer them a follow up appointment in two to four weeks' time to discuss the results with them once available.

Summarise back and conclude

Without going through each and every minute detail, give a brief overview of what you have discussed and agreed upon during your consultation. This will help highlight any miscommunication or misunderstanding that has occurred and may also afford the patient a final chance to raise any further concerns.

At the end of the consultation, it is worth offering the patient some information that they can take away with them. A patient information leaflet is a useful resource that summarises much of what has already been said and may even provide answers to any lingering questions the patient may have.

Doctor:	'So, after the procedure, we'll see you again in about four weeks to see how things are going. Why don't you take this leaflet, it has got all the information we have covered today, and may answer any further questions you may have.'
Mr Evans:	'Thanks, Doctor.'
Doctor:	'If there is anything you would like to discuss before the operation, please get in touch with my secretary and I will get back to you as soon as possible.'
Mr Evans:	'Thank you very much, Doctor.'

FIRST CLINICAL SCENARIO

MRI scanning

Doctors are often asked to explain an investigation. Although it may seem a trivial task, it is a skill that can elude even the most experienced of clinicians. It is important to elicit what the patient understands about the investigation and then address their concerns. Keep your explanations simple and avoid using complex medical terms.

DOCTOR'S BRIEF

You are one of the Foundation Year House Officers in General Practice. One of your patients has attended asking you to explain about an MRI scan he is awaiting.

ACTOR'S BRIEF *(if you are the doctor, please do not read)*

You are Mr Anderson, a 52-year-old IT consultant. You have recently been suffering from headaches which are worse when you are lying in bed, and they are exacerbated by coughing and sneezing. Being quite concerned, you saw your GP who referred you to the Neurologist. Subsequently, you have been told you need an MRI scan. You are quite concerned about this scan, not only because you are afraid of enclosed spaces, but also because you are worried about the possible diagnosis of a brain tumour.

Only volunteer the information about the brain tumour if you feel that the doctor has adequately addressed your concerns about claustrophobia.

SCENARIO WALK-THROUGH

INTRODUCE YOURSELF TO THE PATIENT	*Doctor:*	'Hello, Mr Anderson. My name is Dr Singh. I am one of the doctors here today. How are you doing?'
	Mr A:	*'I'm very well, Doctor.'*
	Doctor:	'That's good to hear. What has brought you to see me today?'
	Mr A:	*'Well, I recently got referred by the hospital for an MRI scan because of these headaches I keep getting.'*
NON-VERBAL CUES TO ENCOURAGE PATIENT TO TALK	*Doctor:*	'Umm hmm.' (*Nodding*)
	Mr A:	*'I was just wondering if I could have a chat with you about the scan as I don't know much about it really. The doctor in the hospital rushed me quite a bit and I couldn't really speak to him about it.'*
	Doctor:	'OK, that's fine. We can have a little chat about MRI scans today and hopefully you will be much clearer about them once we've finished.'
	Mr A:	*'That would be quite useful.'*
CHECK PATIENT'S UNDERSTANDING	*Doctor:*	'So, tell me, what do you already know about MRI scanning?'
	Mr A:	*'Not much to be honest. Just that it makes a detailed scan of my brain.'*
ELICIT PATIENT'S CONCERNS	*Doctor:*	'Yes, that's right, it can actually give us a very detailed picture of the brain, which can be very useful when making a diagnosis.
		'What are your thoughts about it?'
PRIMARY CONCERN	*Mr A:*	*'Well, I've heard it can be quite cramped and noisy in the scanning room. I've got a bit of a phobia of closed spaces.'*
ADDRESS PATIENT'S CONCERNS AND OFFER SOLUTIONS	*Doctor:*	'Yes, that is quite a common concern. I think the first thing to mention is that the scan should not take too long – you will only be there for a short time. There will always be people watching over you from an adjacent room and they will come to your assistance if you need them. You will also be provided with headphones to listen to some soothing music which may help relax you. If things really are too bad, then we can give you some medication to calm your nerves, but only as a last resort.'

Mr A:	'That's sounds reassuring. Hopefully it shouldn't be a problem then.'
Doctor:	'Is there anything else that is worrying you?'
Mr A:	'Well, I'm kind of worried about the results...'
Doctor:	'OK, go on...'
Mr A:	'I'm just really worried whether I've got a tumour causing all this...'
Doctor:	'I appreciate that is a great concern for you. I think it is important to realise that there are many potential causes for the symptoms you are having. The main thing to remember is that you are seeing a Neurologist who is thoroughly investigating you for your symptoms. The MRI scan should go some way in helping us find a cause of your headaches.'
Mr A:	'Yes, that's one way of looking at it I guess...'
Doctor:	'Would you like me to explain a little about how the scanner actually works?'
Mr A:	'OK...'
Doctor:	'MRI stands for magnetic resonance imaging. What this means is that the scan uses magnetic fields to build up a picture of your body. As a result the MRI scan is much safer than a CT scan, which uses X-rays.'
Mr A:	'That's good. So no exposure to harmful beams?'
Doctor:	'Yes, that is the main advantage of MRI. However, as the scan uses magnets, it is important that you do not have any metal objects on you. In addition, we would have to make sure that you do not have a pacemaker or any other metallic implants.'
Mr A:	'No. I am quite well. I am positive that I don't have any metallic objects in me.'
Doctor:	'On the day of the procedure you will see a nurse who will take your details and get you changed into a hospital gown. She will then take you into the room where you will be asked to lie flat. The bed will automatically move into the MRI machine, which looks like a large tumble drier. She will also give you a pair of headphones which should mask out any loud noises that the machine makes.

GIVE INFORMATION
IN BITE-SIZED
PORTIONS

PRE-OP

THE PROCESS		'The whole process should last no longer than about half an hour. The radiographer will be in constant contact with you and may ask you to do some manoeuvres such as holding your breath, to help with getting good quality images.
		'Are you happy with what I have explained so far?'
	Mr A:	*'Yes, pretty much. So how long will it take before I hear my results? Will the radiographer tell me straight away?'*
POST-SCAN PERIOD	Doctor:	'Unfortunately, the radiographer won't be able to discuss the findings with you immediately. The images will need to be checked by a Consultant Radiologist before any results can be given out. I believe that the Consultant Neurologist in the hospital will see you within two to three weeks of the scan and discuss the results with you personally.
OFFER PATIENT INFORMATION LEAFLET		'Why don't you take this leaflet, Mr Anderson? It contains a lot of information about things we've talked about today, and a few extra details about MRI scanners.'
	Mr A:	*'Thank you, Doctor.'*
	Doctor:	'Is there anything else you would like to discuss?'
	Mr A:	*'No, Doctor, you've been great!'*
SUMMARISE BACK	Doctor:	'Just before we finish, is it alright if I briefly go over what we have discussed today?'
	Mr A:	*'Fine.'*
	Doctor:	'You are waiting for an MRI scan to investigate the cause of your headaches. The MRI scanner looks like a large tumble drier and will use a powerful magnet to make detailed images of your body. The whole process should not last more than half an hour and the Consultant will discuss the results with you in two to three weeks' time.'
	Mr A:	*'That sounds about right. Thanks, Doctor. Bye now.'*

CONSULTATION END

SECOND CLINICAL SCENARIO

Tonsillectomy

On occasions, patients consent to having a procedure without fully under-standing its purpose and its risks. It is important to clarify the patient's understanding, and deal with their concerns prior to consenting them for the procedure. Understanding the risks and benefits is key to consenting and it is worth observing your seniors undertaking this process before embarking upon it yourself.

DOCTOR'S BRIEF

You are an ST1 in ENT Surgery. You are doing the pre-op assessment out-patient list today and your next patient is Rachel Taylor, a five-year-old girl, who has attended with her mother. She is due to have a tonsillectomy in a fortnight's time.

ACTOR'S BRIEF *(if you are the doctor, please do not read)*

You are Ms Taylor, a 35-year-old single mother of two. Your child has recently been listed for a tonsillectomy and you think you have come today to sign the consent form for the procedure. You are actually quite concerned about this operation, as you have heard from one of your friends that taking the tonsils out can affect the child's immune system. Furthermore, the thought of your child undergoing a general anaesthetic and 'major surgery' really daunts you.

SCENARIO WALK-THROUGH

INTRODUCE YOURSELF TO THE PATIENT'S RELATIVE	*Doctor:*	'Hello, Ms Taylor. My name is Dr Miller. How are you and your daughter today?'
	Ms Taylor:	*'We're fine thanks, Doctor. Rachel is really looking forward to coming into hospital, aren't you Rachel?'*

(Rachel nods, but is generally preoccupied with the toys in the consulting room)

	Ms Taylor:	*'Yeah . . . she knows she is having her tonsils out, but we haven't really told her too much about it. Just that she'll be staying in hospital overnight.'*
ELICIT RELATIVE'S IDEAS	*Doctor:*	'It is good that she has some understanding of what's going to happen. Ms Taylor, have you been told about the purpose of today's visit?'
	Ms Taylor:	*'Well, I just thought it was for signing the paperwork before the big day.'*
	Doctor:	'Yes, that is one thing we have to do. But today is also about making sure that you are absolutely clear about the procedure and have all your questions answered.'
	Ms Taylor:	*'OK, this should be useful then.'*
ELICIT RELATIVE'S UNDERSTANDING	*Doctor:*	'So, tell me, what do you already understand about the operation?'
	Ms Taylor:	*'I know that they will be putting Rachel to sleep and then the surgeons will be taking out her tonsils. Is that correct?'*
ELICIT RELATIVE'S CONCERNS	*Doctor:*	'That's quite right. Do you have any concerns about this?'
	Ms Taylor:	*'Well, my friends told me that if your tonsils are taken out it will weaken your immune system. Is that right?'*
	Doctor:	'This is a common concern that people have. However, there is no scientific evidence to suggest that people who have their tonsils removed have a weaker immune system. In fact, they have as strong an ability to fight common infections as anyone else.'
	Ms Taylor:	*'Yeah . . . I thought so. Just some of my friends were saying that to me, that's all.'*
ELICIT CONCERNS	*Doctor:*	'Is there anything else worrying you?'

Ms Taylor:	*'Well, she's only five and I'm a bit worried about the whole operation, from the anaesthetic to the operation itself.'*
Doctor:	'Most parents do worry about this especially when their child is so young.'
Ms Taylor:	*'Exactly!'*

PROVIDING REASSURANCE

Doctor:	'Your daughter will be looked after by a highly qualified and specialist team throughout her stay in the hospital, all the way from the ward to the theatre recovery suite. The anaesthetist will be a child specialist, someone who specialises in putting young children to sleep for their operations.'
Ms Taylor:	*'So, the anaesthetist will be a specialist then?'*

PROVIDING REASSURANCE

Doctor:	'Absolutely. Not only that, the Consultant doing the operation has a special interest in children's ears, nose and throat disorders. Also, the theatre recovery staff have all been highly trained in dealing with children's problems.'
Ms Taylor:	*'That's quite reassuring, Doctor.'*

PRE-OP

Doctor:	'Before she comes in for the operation she will need to stop eating for at least six hours prior to the procedure. Seeing as she is having her operation in the morning, it might be an idea to wake her for a midnight snack, and then to keep her fasted from then on.
PAUSE	
	'She will be taken from the ward to the pre-op room where she will meet an anaesthetist. They will pass a small plastic tube into her hand and give her some oxygen to breath. They will put her to sleep and allow the surgeon to begin. Is that OK?'
Ms Taylor:	*'Yes.'*

THE OPERATION

Doctor:	'During the operation, the surgeon will locate and remove Rachel's tonsils. It is quite a short procedure and should last only 20 minutes.'
Ms Taylor:	*'Really? As quick as that?'*

POST-OP

Doctor:	'After the operation, Rachel will be transferred to one of the wards to recover. The nurse will be closely

		monitoring her during this time. The Consultant will later review her and make sure she is well enough to go home.
	Ms Taylor:	*'OK ... Will she be in pain when she wakes up?'*
IMMEDIATE POST-OP SIDE EFFECTS	Doctor:	'After the operation, she might experience a little pain, but we will give her regular pain relief for this.
		'In terms of eating, many people suggest initially providing a diet of soft jelly, ice cream or soup. If she is able to tolerate this you can then consider introducing solids.
	PAUSE	
		'It might be advisable that Rachel takes about two weeks off school and avoids any strenuous activities. This is to allow for her throat to heal.'
	Ms Taylor:	*'OK, that's quite useful advice.'*
RISK AND COMPLICATIONS	Doctor:	'That's good. However, although this is a safe operation, with any procedure there are risks and complications to be aware of. The main thing to watch out for is bleeding and infection at the site of the operation.'
	Ms Taylor:	*'Oh really! That sounds worrying.'*
	Doctor:	'The risk of this happening is quite rare (less than 1%). However, it is common to see slight bleeding persisting for up to two weeks.'
	Ms Taylor:	*'So, what should I do if I notice a lot of blood?'*
	Doctor:	'Try to remain calm, and bring her to A&E straight away. One of the ENT specialists will then see her. In most cases, the bleeding stops by itself and we just need to monitor the situation. In a small number of cases the patient may need to go back to theatre to stop the bleeding, but like I said this is quite rare. In any case our specialists are highly trained to deal with any of the complications I have described to you.'
	Ms Taylor:	*'OK.'*
	Doctor:	'In terms of infection, if you notice that Rachel develops a fever or sore throat within the next two

weeks, bring her back as she may need to have a course of antibiotics.'

Ms Taylor: 'OK then. That's very helpful.'

FOLLOW-UP

Doctor: 'After about two months, the Consultant would like to review Rachel in outpatients to make sure she is doing well, and that her symptoms have resolved.'

Ms Taylor: 'That's great, Doctor. You've clarified so much for me today!

SUMMARISE BACK

Doctor: 'Before you leave, I just want to make sure that I have been clear in my explanation. To summarise, Rachel is due for an operation to remove her tonsils. It is a common procedure and will be performed by one of our specialists. She will have to fast from midnight before the operation. She will later be seen by a specialist anaesthetist who will put her to sleep before the surgeons remove her tonsils.

PAUSE

'After the operation she may feel a bit sore and notice slight bleeding. However, if she develops a temperature, sore throat or excessive bleeding then we may need to see assess her in A&E.

OFFER PATIENT INFORMATION LEAFLET

'Here is a short leaflet about tonsillectomy summarising what we have discussed today. It has a lot of information and helpful tips for you. It may be an idea to read through this before we see you again.'

Ms Taylor: 'Thanks, Doctor. I'll see you on the day.'

Doctor: 'Take care.'

CONSULTATION END

CHAPTER 7

Intra-professional communication

As a junior doctor, you will be spending a large proportion of your time communicating with fellow doctors, be it on ward rounds, in A&E or simply when lounging around in the doctors' mess. These conversations may involve discussions about day-to-day activities, politics or one's social life. However, there are times when conversations with colleagues have a greater importance, especially when discussing patients' illnesses, investigations and their management. Hence, it is of vital importance to use good communication to ensure that miscommunication does not take place.

Although you will be more commonly interacting with doctors of a similar grade to yourself, you will frequently be required to speak with colleagues of a more senior rank. On occasions you may be asked to discuss a case with a Consultant Radiologist when making a specific request for an investigation, or to make a referral to the relevant Registrar on call, for a specialist opinion. Although these situations may at first appear quite daunting, with the correct application of communication skills and medical knowledge you will be able to negotiate competently through this task.

From time to time your intra-professional communications will be tested by situations that may not be clinical in nature, e.g. something as benign as swapping a shift or organising annual leave. Other times, it may tested by something far more complex, such as a discussion about a colleague's ability to perform competently. In such circumstances, the challenge will lie in your ability to gain the trust of your colleague, and to maintain rapport with them while negotiating an amicable solution that does not put the safety of the patient at risk.

Communicating with colleagues

The way doctors communicate with each other differs greatly from how they communicate with patients. In relation to the patient, the doctor's overriding objective is to deliver safe, effective and appropriate care whilst communicating this in a simple and jargon-free manner. Between doctors, there exists a commonality of generic skills and medical knowledge, which in theory should make communication easier. However in practice, intra-professional communication is often quite challenging, especially so when the subject matter is of a sensitive nature.

The consultation: intra-professional communication

It is likely that in the clinical setting you will have already established rapport with a number of colleagues from your day-to-day encounters with them. With such colleagues, it is unnecessary to go through the rigmarole of reintroducing oneself and re-establishing rapport. On the other hand, be wary of trivialising the conversation by being too casual or informal in your discussions with them. It is important, particularly when talking about sensitive issues, to maintain a sense of professionalism and accountability, as this will add an element of seriousness to the conversation.

Often, the introductory statement you use will set the tone for the rest of the conversation. Imagine the reaction if you were to burst into your Consultant's room with a list of demands in an accusatory way.

Doctor: 'I am glad I finally caught you! I've come to address the long hours I've been working recently. I'm sure you know that the European Working Time Directive has come into force and my union is telling me that my rota is currently illegal!'

Consultant: 'How dare you burst into my room and threaten me!'

Such a start to a conversation will give rise to ill feeling, which will not bode well for the rest of the meeting. Even if the meeting concerns a legitimate disagreement or grievance, every effort should be made to maintain a courteous and professional approach to facilitate a positive outcome.

Doctor: 'Hello, Dr Smith. Thank you for agreeing to see me at such short notice.'

Consultant: 'Oh, that's OK. Now tell me, what can I do for you?'

Doctor: 'Well, it's about these past two weeks we've had on the ward . . .'

Consultant: 'Oh, it's been horrendous hasn't it? I've never known it to be so busy. I really appreciate your hard work in that time. Even I've had to stay behind because of the long ward rounds, just to make sure my clinics and paperwork are completed . . .'

In situations where you are meeting a fellow colleague for the first time, it is important to maintain the formalities of the proceedings by stating your name, designation and the purpose of the conversation. Apart from being courteous, it is also important in medico-legal terms as it helps establish who you are, what relationship you have with the patient and who to return to for future reference.

Establishing the problem

You may find yourself in a situation or scenario where it is necessary to try to understand the problems and difficulties a colleague is facing. In such cases you should try to be empathic and sensitive when attempting to raise the subject with them. Use open questions so that you appear non-judgemental and non-accusatory. By doing this, your colleague will feel more at ease with you and be more prone to discuss any personal matters that are concerning them.

Doctor: 'Hey John, I've noticed you've been turning up late for work every day this week. I just wanted you to know that it's gone too far now and I've had enough of having to cover your bleep and see your patients.'

Colleague: 'If you haven't already heard, my dad's just been told he's got lung cancer and has only a few months to live. I've spent the past two weeks trying to sort out his affairs and cope with the shock of it all.'

Doctor: 'Oh . . . I had no idea . . . errr . . .'

Colleague: 'Forget it. You've said enough.'

Expressing empathy

Whilst doctors are very good at expressing empathy towards their patients, they often fail to do so when dealing with fellow professionals. Most doctors will admit that they are overworked and lack time for recreational activities but, because it is expected to be part of their job, most doctors simply 'grin and bear it'.

Unfortunately, this widely held belief often disregards an individual's personal circumstances. One may be quick to pass judgement upon a previously hardworking and diligent doctor, who is now repeatedly attending work late, as being inconsiderate and irresponsible, whereas providing a sympathetic ear may help reveal whatever personal difficulties they are facing. Use active listening and empathic non-verbal cues to help you establish the problem and your colleague's perspective on the matter.

Doctor: 'Hi John, how are you doing?'

Colleague: 'Up and down. I'm finding it hard to focus on my work, to be honest.'

Doctor: 'I'm sorry to hear that. Do you want to talk about it?'

Colleague: 'Well . . . I'm having a few problems at home. My dad's not well . . .'

Doctor:	'Really? I am so sorry to hear that.'
Colleague:	'Yeah. It's been a difficult few weeks. I have to pass by my dad's place before I come to work to make sure he's OK. I am finding hard to juggle everything.'
Doctor:	'Do you want to discuss this in private?'

Suggest possible solutions

By being empathic you are likely to have elicited the crux of the matter in an amicable and non-confrontational way. After digesting all the facts you should now be able to suggest a few possible solutions to ease your colleague's predicament. Naturally, the details will need to be tailored to the problems or circumstances that they find themselves in.

Doctor:	'Have you thought about taking some time off from work to sort out these problems?'
Colleague:	'Yeah, I have but I think that I have run out of annual leave.'
Doctor:	'What about if we swap a few shifts?'
Colleague:	'I can't do that. You are already covering me enough and I don't want to overburden you anymore.'
Doctor:	'OK. What if we go to your training supervisor and try to arrange some compassionate leave. I don't think it will be a problem to organise given your situation . . .'

Negotiating

You may find yourself on occasions being asked to undertake responsibilities that are not suitable for your level, or being requested to regularly work beyond your contracted hours. Although it is easy to get intimidated and railroaded into following an unreasonable course of action, it is important that you get your point across in a polite and professional manner. This will hopefully allow both parties to negotiate an amicable solution.

Doctor:	'I've been told that my rota has changed and I am going to have to work two weekends in a row, on call!'
Consultant:	'Yes, unfortunately that's the case. One of the doctors has fallen sick again.'
Doctor:	'I think it is unfair that I wasn't told this before and am now expected to cover at the last minute. Besides, that would make my rota illegal according to the European Working Time Directive!'
Consultant:	'Well, that's the way it is unfortunately!'
Doctor:	'My union will be hearing about this!'

Whilst in principle the junior doctor is correct that the new hours will not comply with the European Working Time Directive, their approach has left no room for negotiation. In addition, they have failed to appreciate the Consultant's perspective and reasons for this decision. Even if the outcome was that the doctor could not, or would not, work for two consecutive weekends, their abrupt and brash manner is unlikely to be received well by their Consultant. Consider this alternative approach:

Doctor:	'Hello, Dr Johnson. I understand you wanted to talk to me about working another weekend after this one?'
Consultant:	'Yes, I understand that this is not an ideal situation but there is a reason I have asked for this . . .'
Doctor:	'It sounds like things are quite difficult at the moment.'
Consultant:	'Indeed. Unfortunately someone called in sick again and a gap has arisen. I was hoping you would be able to help. I would of course make sure that you aren't faced with a similar scenario again and would also give you a day off in lieu after the second weekend.'
Doctor:	'I understand your predicament. I would be happy to help. It is just that I am already booked for a commitment on that Sunday which I can't cancel at this late stage. However I would be able to cover on Saturday.'
Consultant:	'That would be a massive help for me. However, that still leaves Sunday though . . .'
Doctor:	'I could bleep some of the other SHOs on the firms and see whether any of them can cover the Sunday.'
Consultant:	'Oh, thank you for agreeing to help out. I do really appreciate your help.'

In this example, the junior doctor has utilised good negotiation skills to help achieve a cordial solution. The doctor appreciated the Consultant's dilemma and incorporated this in their plan of action. Apart from maintaining a good relationship with the Consultant, he has managed to negotiate time off in lieu for his efforts.

Examples of intra-professional conversations

What we have discussed so far will provide you with a good grounding in intra-professional communication. However, the framework will need to be tailored depending on the seniority or speciality of the doctor you are in conversation with. It must be appreciated that communicating with a Foundation Year doctor will be quite different to a conversation with a Consultant. Equally, referring a patient to a radiologist for an inpatient ultrasound-guided biopsy will be quite different than when referring a patient to the general surgeons for an emergency laparotomy. The following section will give you some pointers to consider when faced with different circumstances.

Communicating with a Consultant

The Consultant is the head of the firm and is usually the equivalent of your 'boss'. Your relationship with them will, therefore, be more formal in nature and your language and approach should reflect this. However, more often than not, they will also be your clinical supervisor providing you with pastoral support and care should you face any problems or difficulties. In these circumstances conversations can be candid and honest in nature.

Consultants are extremely busy people and do not appreciate unplanned, spontaneous visits. It is therefore better to book your meeting beforehand through an appointment via their secretary. You may wish to plan your meeting ahead by noting down important points that you want to discuss.

When you commence your meeting with your Consultant, do not be fazed or perturbed if your Consultant is constantly interrupted by phone calls and bleeps, or leaves prematurely. A Consultant is often laboured with duties and responsibilities in addition to their clinical duties of care.

Communicating with a senior member of the team (SHO, Registrar)

Clinical firms consist of a hierarchy that includes a Consultant, Registrar, Senior House Officer and Foundation Year House Officer. You are likely to develop close working relationships with the less-senior members of your firm as you will be working together for the bulk of your clinical attachment. This may create an informal atmosphere which should facilitate easy communication with your colleagues. However, on the other hand, be wary of appearing unprofessional in front of patients or allied health staff.

When communicating with colleagues in your team, it is likely that simple problems and complaints will be dealt with informally. If, however, you feel that the seriousness of the situation warrants a more formal setting, you should indicate this prior to your meeting.

On occasions, you may be asked by a senior member of your team to perform duties or tasks that you feel are beyond your capabilities, such as a Foundation Year House Officer doctor performing a lumbar puncture or inserting an arterial line unsupervised. Sometimes you may be requested inappropriately to cover a senior's absence due to their attendance at a course or postgraduate examination. Whatever the reason, irrespective of your rapport with the firm, if you do not feel comfortable with such responsibilities you should make your feelings clear and explain why you are concerned.

Senior SHO: 'I'm teaching medical students at the medical school today,

	but Mr Jones needs a central line inserted this afternoon. I won't be around, so could you put it in?'
FY1:	'I've not done any central lines before.'
Senior SHO:	'What? I did 10 when I was a House Officer. They're dead easy. You saw one in theatre the other day, didn't you?'
FY1:	'Yes, but . . .'
Senior SHO:	'Don't you know the old adage of "see one, do one, teach one"?'
FY1:	'Yes, but . . .'
Senior SHO:	'There's nothing to it. Just find the internal jugular with the Doppler probe – you can't miss it, insert the needle, flashback, guide-wire, dilator, line, stitch. Piece of cake. Trust me you're good, you'll have no problem. I'll see you tomorrow then. If you get stuck there's a good diagram in the back of baby Kumar & Clark! I'll be back tomorrow morning then.'
FY1:	'Err . . . OK.'

Imagine the potential risk to the patient if this doctor decided, under peer pressure, to go ahead despite not being adequately trained or competent. Bear in mind that in the event of a disaster, blaming a colleague would not be an adequate defence. Now consider an alternative approach by a more assertive doctor:

FY1:	'I've not done any central lines before.'
Senior SHO:	'What? I did 10 when I was a House Officer. They're dead easy. You saw one in theatre the other day, didn't you?'
FY1:	'Yes, but I have not performed any under supervision. I need to be supervised in order to do it.'
Senior SHO:	'There's nothing to it. Just find the internal jugular with the Doppler probe – you can't miss it, insert the needle, flashback, guide-wire, dilator, line, stitch. Piece of cake. Trust me – you're good, you'll have no problem. I'll see you tomorrow then.'
FY1:	'No, I'm sorry, but I will not do it without supervision. I don't feel that I have adequate training to do this on my own and I do not want to cause any harm to the patient. I realise that you have this teaching session which I know is very important and I don't want you to miss it. Perhaps, you could arrange with one of the other senior SHOs who have done central lines before to supervise me. I think Jeff's around today and not too busy?'

Senior SHO: 'Right. OK, I'll speak to Jeff and ask him.'

FY1:   'Thanks. Let me know once it's confirmed. I'll go ahead and provisionally book the Doppler and make sure we have all the equipment on the ward. I'll also make sure I clean up afterwards.'

Senior SHO: 'Alright, fine. I'll let you know what's happening.'

The overriding issue here is patient safety and the doctor is perfectly within their rights to refuse to carry out the procedure even if it means their colleague missing out on teaching. However, application of the principles discussed earlier has enabled an amicable outcome to be negotiated. Again, this example demonstrates empathy in understanding the situation of the colleague, negotiating and finally reaching a mutually acceptable plan. The doctor has also managed to seize an excellent learning opportunity by not simply refusing, but agreeing to perform the procedure under supervision.

Communicating with other specialties

The responsibility for communicating with other doctors from different specialties will often fall upon the shoulder of the most junior members of the team. This is often a cause of great anxiety as it may mean having to face a barrage of unpleasant questions from a hostile Registrar or SHO. Unfortunately, this is very much part and parcel of your job but hopefully it will become less threatening with experience and knowledge.

Conversations with other specialties usually take place in the context of a simple telephone call. Your ability to communicate clearly and concisely, emphasising the key points, is therefore paramount. There are several things which can be done to reduce the unease associated with these scenarios, in accordance with the framework described earlier.

Firstly, it is a good idea to summarise in the patient's notes the salient points of the patient's history, working diagnosis, recent investigations and treatments to date. Your documentation will not only act as a prompt when talking with your colleague, but also provide written evidence that a handover of care has taken place.

Secondly, empathise with the receiving speciality. Try to put yourself in their position and ask yourself, *'If someone was making this referral to me what information would I like to know?'*

Lastly, when referring, you should try to be as concise as possible, avoiding any unnecessary details. Do not waste valuable time speaking about irrelevant family history of the patient in an acute emergency. Consider the following example:

Doctor:	'Hi, I'm Phil, one of the surgical FY1s. I wonder if I could ask you to review one of my patients.'
Resp. SPR:	'Yes, I'm listening.'
Doctor:	'I have a patient who is breathless, and my Consultant wants a respiratory review.'
Resp. SPR:	'So . . . who is this patient?'
Doctor:	'Errr . . . one minute . . . the name is . . . Julie Watson.'
Resp. SPR:	'And how old is she?'
Doctor:	'Erm . . . around 80, I think.'
Resp. SPR:	'And what's wrong with her?'
Doctor:	'Well . . . that's why we want you to see her.'
Resp. SPR:	'For God's sake, I mean is she breathless, wheezy, coughing, what is the complaint?'
Doctor:	'Oh . . . she had a hemicolectomy two days ago – and on the ward round today she was breathless.'
Resp. SPR:	'Right. So have you done any investigations? Do you have any ideas what's going on?'
Doctor:	'Well you're the medic – we were hoping you could help . . .'
Resp. SPR:	'I don't believe what I'm hearing! What does her chest sound like? Any wheezes or crackles? Have you done an X-ray? Is she tachycardic? Does she have a cough or fever?'
Doctor:	'Err . . .'
Resp. SPR:	'Have you done an ECG? Blood tests? Blood gases?'
Doctor:	'Err . . .'
Resp. SPR:	'Right. Go away, examine the patient, do some blood tests, a chest X-ray and an ECG and THEN, if you can't figure it out, call me back. Goodbye!'

Unfortunately, this is quite a common occurrence in many hospitals. Looking at it from the respiratory Registrar's perspective, it is not unreasonable to expect the referring doctor to have some knowledge about the patient's presenting complaint, to have done some basic investigations and to have made a possible working diagnosis. By performing relevant investigations your task in referring the patient will be made much easier.

Another mistake made by junior doctors when in trouble is to try to deflect responsibility for the referral back to their own Consultant stating that *'they requested the referral'*. Whilst this may be true it provides no extra useful information towards the patient's care and may irk your senior colleague further.

Communicating with a poorly performing colleague

During your professional career, you may find yourself in a situation where you are working with a poorly performing colleague. Although thankfully uncommon, when it presents it may endanger patients' lives and safety. Such scenarios often pose challenges to one's own communication skills in managing the dilemma.

Underperforming colleagues are often difficult to identify as they may excel in covering up their mistakes, and may be exposed only after gross misconduct, such as putting a patient's life at risk. Early signs of underperformance may include simple drug errors, arriving late to work, not completing their duties or simply being poorly communicative.

However, it is important not to jump to conclusions about a colleague's performance. If you have noticed simple errors you should bring them to their attention in a non-judgemental manner. Being critical may inadvertently affect your future working relationship with them and make them feel that they are being constantly watched. If despite your advice they persist in their behaviour, you have a duty of care for the patients to intervene.

Doctor: 'David, that's the third time you've prescribed 125 milligrams of digoxin instead of 125 micrograms! I'm fed up with covering for your mistakes. Unless you get your act together, I will seriously consider going to the Consultant and telling him what a useless doctor you are.'

Colleague: 'What mistakes? I don't know what you talking about.'

Doctor: 'I've counted three drug errors in one week and that's three too many!'

Colleague: 'Who appointed you as my guardian angel? If I did make these mistakes why didn't you just tell me before? All I did was forget the 'c' in mcg. Its not such a big deal as the nurses know what doses to give.'

Doctor: 'It's completely unacceptable and no excuse can justify it.'

Colleague: 'You have no clue what I've been through this week! Besides, this mistake won't happen again!'

As the above example highlights, you should not be too hasty in confronting your colleague with 'hard facts'. You are more likely to resolve the problem if you adopt a more empathic and non-accusatory tone. This will allow your colleague to feel comfortable with you when discussing the reasons behind their actions.

Doctor: 'I feel that you're not your usual self; you're normally so enthusiastic and full of energy. Is everything OK?'

Colleague: 'I'm fine. Everything's fine.'

Doctor:	'I am just a bit worried. The nurse pointed out that you made a few mistakes on a drug chart, so I just wanted to make sure everything was alright?'
Colleague:	'Oh, you mean the digoxin doses? I remember . . . that was simply an oversight.'
Doctor:	'Well, you've been with the firm for a few months now and you have never made that mistake before. I am just a bit worried that whatever is on your mind is beginning to affect patient care.'
Colleague:	'Look, I am sorry. My wife had a miscarriage last week and my mind has been elsewhere.'
Doctor:	'I am so sorry. I did not know that was the case. Do you want to go somewhere quiet to discuss this?'

Depending on the situation, your colleague may need to be directed to their educational supervisor, the sub-dean of the hospital or, if available a welfare officer who can provide support and advice. This will ensure that your colleague will receive the correct supervision and support to guide them through their difficult period.

When offering advice to seek help on behalf of your colleague, do not forget to explore their ideas and concerns about your suggestions. Your colleague may feel betrayed if you were to go to a senior staff member without their consent after they had confided in you.

Once you have agreed on a plan of action you should reflect this back to your colleague and ensure that they understand and agree with it. This will give them an opportunity to raise any concerns about the proposal.

Doctor:	'I am sorry to hear that your wife had a miscarriage. Have you thought of talking to your Consultant about taking compassionate leave?'
Colleague:	'Yeah. I've tried speaking to my Registrar as well as my Consultant, but they are not having any of it. Apparently we have no cover for next week's nights.'
Doctor:	'What about speaking to the Deanery about it?'
Colleague:	'Yes. I have thought about it but I don't want this to affect my career.'
Doctor:	'Well, I am on annual leave next week. How about if I cover you next week and you have that week off? We can always sort out the details later on.'
Colleague:	'Oh, that's so kind. That will give me some time with my family . . .'

FIRST SCENARIO

Lack of senior support

Junior doctors have always had to work in tough, fast-paced and unforgiving environments. In recent years the emphasis on patient safety has led to a change in the training of junior doctors. No longer is it acceptable practice for them to work unsupervised and for long extended hours. However, on occasions where firms are short staffed, it is still expected that doctors will fill in shifts and cover for gaps in the rota. Short staffing and poor senior support leads to unchecked errors, mistakes in management, poor working conditions and can even cause ill health in doctors.

When discussing rota concerns with seniors, it is important to avoid being confrontational and obstinate in your conduct. This is unlikely to improve things and will damage intra-professional relationships in the long run. A polite, formal approach, taking the opportunity to establish rapport and to understand the point of view of your senior, will give rise to a productive dialogue and will increase your chances of reaching an agreeable plan.

DOCTOR'S BRIEF

You are the Foundation Year House Officer in Care of the Elderly Medicine. You work in an extremely busy department under one of the Consultants, Dr Hendry. You are in the middle of a particularly busy period and have now worked for two weeks without an SHO or fellow Foundation Year House Officer. Your Registrar is usually away at clinic, teaching or studying for his Master's degree.

You are regularly starting early and finishing late and feel that due to your inexperience, patient safety is at risk. Additionally, you cannot remember the last time you were able to take a lunch break and constantly feel tired and drained. You are also concerned that you are unable to attend your time-tabled teaching sessions due to there being no cover on the wards. You have requested a meeting with your Consultant to discuss the situation.

ACTOR'S BRIEF *(if you are the doctor, please do not read)*

You are Dr Hendry, Consultant in Care of the Elderly Medicine. You are aware that it has been a particularly busy time for the hospital and you have had a large number of acute admissions. Unfortunately, your SHO has had to take time off due to a family bereavement and despite your efforts, medical staffing has been unable to provide a replacement or locum. Your Registrar's contract guarantees him weekly study leave for his Master's degree and you have signed an agreement with the medical school that allows him to teach on a regular basis. To top it all off, your ward is short staffed.

You have been particularly impressed by your Foundation Year doctor, who you feel is taking on the additional responsibility and workload well. You feel he exceeds expectations and are happy at the way in which he seems to be managing the patients on the ward. You are aware that he is often staying late although you feel it is good experience for him as a doctor.

He has now asked to speak to you in person and you suspect it is with regard to the increased workload and long hours. Although you would like to help, you are struggling to find a solution. You are open to any reasonable suggestions and are happy to take them up with hospital management. However, you will not take kindly to being pressurised and will get irritated if anyone tries to blackmail or threaten you.

You do not have authority to recruit staff although you are good friends with the other medical Consultants who often seem to have SHOs with very little work to do.

SCENARIO WALK-THROUGH

INTRODUCE YOURSELF IN A NON-CONFRONTATIONAL MANNER	*Doctor:*	'Hello, Dr Hendry. Thank you for taking time to see me at such short notice today. How are you?'
	Dr H:	*'That's OK. How are things with you?'*
ESTABLISH RAPPORT	*Doctor:*	'I'm fine, thank you. I was wondering if I could discuss a few concerns I've been having lately?'
	Dr H:	*'Of course. Fire away.'*
ELICIT IDEAS	*Doctor:*	'I'm sure you're aware of the recent busy period we've had on this firm?'
	Dr H:	*'Absolutely. It's good experience for you though. I'm sure you are seeing a lot of interesting cases. You're doing very well, might I add.'*
DEMONSTRATE UNDERSTANDING AND SHOW EMPATHY	*Doctor:*	'Thanks. It must also be quite tough on you as well with the pressure from the bed managers to free up beds on the wards?'
	Dr H:	*'You're absolutely right. I hope that it's not causing you too much of a problem?'*
APPROPRIATELY DISCUSS CONCERNS	*Doctor:*	'Well, to be honest things have been especially tough for the past two weeks since the other SHO left.'
	Dr H:	*'I know. I'm afraid it is a bit tough. But like I said, you're doing very well, and I'm sure you're learning lots.'*
	Doctor:	'I am learning new things every day. However, I do have a few concerns regarding the situation.
	PAUSE	
		'Since the other SHO left, I'm having to come in two hours earlier and also I'm leaving work around two hours later each day. At times I'm also going without a lunch break because it has just been too busy.'
	Dr H:	*'I'm sorry to hear that. It reminds me of when I was a House Officer. In those days of course, we regularly worked 100 hours a week as part of the job!'*
DO NOT BE INTIMIDATED TO PLAY DOWN YOUR CONCERNS	*Doctor:*	'I fully appreciate your point. However, I feel that I am not able to do my job to the best of my ability and this may compromise patient care. Your support has been great but you have other commitments which

often take you away from the ward for long periods and I am worried that I may make mistakes.

PAUSE

I am so tired and towards the end of the day, with no breaks, I am having trouble concentrating . . .'

Dr H: *'I see . . . We are trying our best to get help at short notice but it is a bit more difficult than I had anticipated. For what it's worth, I think you are doing a grand job.'*

SUGGEST ACTIONS/ PROACTIVE APPROACH

Doctor: 'I was just wondering whether it is possible to arrange a locum to help fill the gaps?'

Dr H: *'Hmm. I have already tried that with medical staffing, but unfortunately I have had no response to date.'*

Doctor: 'Well, I was hoping the Registrar could make himself available a little bit more. He is very helpful and we get along well. I understand he has other commitments but I thought . . . maybe for a short time until we're past this period?'

Dr H: *'I'm afraid not. He booked his study leave for an upcoming exam a while ago and has his university teaching commitments.'*

Doctor: 'Perhaps we could borrow an SHO from one of the other medical firms?'

Dr H: *'I haven't tried that yet. But now that you have mentioned it, I am sure there are other teams that are not as busy as we are. I will have to speak to one of their Consultants and see if they're agreeable. We could raise this at the next departmental meeting.'*

PROACTIVE IN EXECUTING PLAN

Doctor: 'That sounds like a good idea. I wonder if there's anything I could do to facilitate it? I'm happy to help in any way that I can.'

Dr H: *'No, that's fine. I'm having a medical meeting this afternoon, I will raise it then. Is there anything else you'd like to discuss?'*

Doctor: 'No, thank you. I hope things go well in your meeting and that you are able to raise support for one of the other SHOs to help us out. I am sure that by doing this things will be a lot easier for us all.'

	Dr H. '*Yes, exactly.*'

THANK COLLEAGUE. CLOSE

Doctor: 'Thank you so much for sparing this time to see me. I am really grateful for your support.'

CONSULTATION END

Poorly performing colleague

Most doctors will encounter colleagues who, on occasions, do not work to an acceptable standard. This may be accompanied by a change in mood, character or demeanour, which may indicate that something is amiss.

It is all too easy to complain and pour scorn on a poorly performing colleague without exploring the reasons why. The medical profession is tough, and most doctors are keen to put on a brave face even when they should be taking time off work due to illness or personal problems.

When having a discussion with a poorly performing colleague, it is important to aim to maintain good rapport in order to avoid any strain on your working relationships. Be sensitive and non-judgemental in your approach. Try to elicit your colleague's own perspective about what is going on and offer support whenever possible. However, if your colleague's actions are putting patients' lives at risk then you will be duty bound to involve other parties, such as the Consultant.

DOCTOR'S BRIEF

You are the Foundation Year House Officer in General Surgery. For the past three days, your fellow Foundation Year colleague, Dr Tom Wilkinson, has been arriving late to work looking dishevelled and tired. During yesterday's Consultant ward round you were blamed for several errors which you know to be the fault of Tom. Despite him arriving at work late, he has been leaving early and you are becoming annoyed at his lack of commitment and silly mistakes. You are also becoming fed up with having to make excuses for him and covering his bleep.

This recent change in behaviour is completely out of character for Tom, who until now has maintained very high standards of professionalism and clinical care. You have decided to have a conversation with him during lunch to discuss your concerns.

ACTOR'S BRIEF (if you are the doctor, please do not read)

You are Dr Tom Wilkinson, a Foundation Year doctor on the surgical firm. Four days ago your mother was involved in a road traffic accident. She is currently stable but in a critical condition at an intensive therapy unit close to your parents' home, 100 miles away. You are visiting her on a daily basis and in order to do this you have to take a two-hour train journey each way.

You are also spending the night at your family home to care for your father, who suffered a stroke two years ago and has impaired mobility. However, because you have already used up your annual leave, you are unable to take any more time off.

You are also an extremely private person and do not wish to discuss this with anyone at work. You are concerned that your Consultant will find out and may comment about it in your end of year review, affecting your career progression through surgery.

You have agreed to meet your colleague at lunch but will be extremely reluctant to disclose any information as you are not sure if your colleague will keep this information private. You are aware, however, that you have made a few mistakes recently and wish to explain these mistakes without jeopardising the good standing you are known to have.

SCENARIO WALK-THROUGH

INTRODUCE YOURSELF IN A NON-CONFRONTATIONAL MANNER	*Doctor:*	'Hi, Tom – how have you been today?'
	Tom:	*'OK, I guess.'*
ESTABLISH RAPPORT	*Doctor:*	'I think the wards have been busy this week. What do you think?'
	Tom:	*'Maybe a little bit. Sorry – did you want to talk to me about something? I have to rush off soon . . .'*
ESTABLISH THE PROBLEM	*Doctor:*	'Sorry, I don't mean to hold you back. I just wanted to talk to you as I've noticed you've not been yourself for the past few days. I was wondering if anything is the matter?'
	Tom:	*'No, I'm fine. I've just been a bit busy with other things.'*
	Doctor:	'Well, you've been more than just a few minutes late on several occasions this week. You look really tired and not your usual smart self.
	PAUSE	
DO NOT BE ACCUSATORY. USE EMPATHIC SKILLS		'What's really worrying me is that you've made a few mistakes that have been completely out of character. Even the nurses have been noticing it.'
	Tom:	*'Look, nothing's wrong. I'm just having a bad week. Everyone makes mistakes.'*
	Doctor:	'I accept that everyone makes mistakes. I just feel that there is something going on which is not allowing you to focus like you normally would.
	PAUSE	
		'I know it can be difficult to talk about these things. But if you don't try to sort things out now, I'm worried it could start affecting patients and the Consultants will notice.'
	Tom:	*'Look – my mum's in hospital and there's no one to look after my dad. They live in Kettering. I need to visit my mum and look after my dad and get back here for work every single day.'*
DEMONSTRATE EMPATHY AND OFFER SUPPORT	*Doctor:*	'I'm very sorry to hear that. It must be really hard for you.

PAUSE

> 'I'm here to offer you support. Why don't you inform the Consultant? I am sure he can arrange for you to have some time off.'

Tom: *'I'd rather not do that. I don't want the Consultant thinking I'm not committed and not give me a good reference. I'd rather show my face on the wards.*

'Look, I'd really appreciate it if for the next few days I could leave straight after the ward round to be with my mum and that you wouldn't let anyone know?'

MAINTAIN PROFESSIONAL STANDARDS. STAND FIRM REGARDING CONCERNS

Doctor: 'Well, I wish I could help but I don't think it's fair on the patients.

'I know that you have a lot to deal with but what you have been doing for the past week, with the mistakes and all that, could really have harmed someone. Don't you think that it would be more damaging to your career if something bad happened?'

Tom: *'I don't know. I am worried about my reference.'*

Doctor: 'I think that the hospital and seniors would be very understanding. They know how committed you are; you've shown that since you started this job. They are not going to look unfavourably at you taking some time off in this difficult situation.'

Tom: *'Maybe you are right. I think that I need to sort this all out. Don't I?'*

OFFER USEFUL SUGGESTIONS

Doctor: 'How about if I come with you and back you up? I'm happy to put in a positive word for you. I really think it would be better if we let someone know now.'

Tom: *'Would you really?'*

AGREE ON PLAN

Doctor: 'Of course. I think we should arrange to see someone today so that this can be sorted. That way you can get away sooner and I can make sure that I have enough support on the wards. Agreed?'

CONCLUDE

'Tom: *'Agreed. Thanks.'*

CONSULTATION END

Setting the scene

Informing a patient that a mistake has taken place is similar to how one goes about breaking bad news. You should set the scene and surroundings accordingly and seek out a quiet room to have your discussion. It is also important to allow for ample uninterrupted time to discuss the matter thoroughly and answer any questions.

Introducing yourself and establishing rapport

Although a mistake has occurred, do not feel hesitant in trying to establish rapport with the patient through professional etiquette and a polite manner. Rapport building in this situation will help maintain a relationship of trust and confidence between yourself and the patient and will allow for a frank discussion.

Establishing patient's awareness

Assuming the patient is as yet unaware of the mistake, you should begin by asking an open question. You may wish to ask the patient about how they feel, or how they view their care in hospital. The patient's response to this question may give you an insight into their level of satisfaction with the service up until now, or if they have any suspicions as to whether anything has gone wrong. It will also allow you to determine their mood, which will help guide you through the rest of the consultation.

Even if the patient seems content and happy, you should still try to establish whether they have any concerns or worries. Apart from acting as a warning shot to the patient, it may help reveal any underlying anxieties they may have. Often when mistakes occur, patients may have an inkling that something is amiss by the change in behaviour of the staff towards them or from inadvertently overhearing a medical conversation. Consider the following example:

Doctor: 'Do you have any concerns or worries regarding your treatment?'

Mr Simon: 'Well, it's just something I heard the nurses mention. It's probably nothing but I can't help thinking about it.'

Doctor: 'Well, I am interested in knowing any concern you may have, no matter how small. Please don't hesitate in letting us know about anything that is worrying you.'

Mr Simon: 'Hmmm . . . it's just that I was given a different drug today. I asked the nurse why and they said that the doctor had changed it in the morning but I hadn't been told. I thought "no, that can't be right", as I didn't see the doctor

CHAPTER 8

Inter-professional communication

Although doctors spend most of their time with fellow colleagues, relationships with other health professionals are equally as important. Doctors, in fact, may spend only a few minutes of the day interacting with their patients whilst other staff members, such as occupational therapists, physiotherapists, dieticians and ward sisters, may spend longer periods with them. This extra time may provide them with valuable additional information about the patient which may contribute to their overall treatment. Hence, good inter-professional communication between doctors and other health professionals is essential to maintain a high standard of patient care.

In days gone by, a paternalistic approach was commonplace in the medical profession with the doctor's opinion being final. Communication between doctors and nurses would often be lopsided with the doctor usually dictating what should be done. Thankfully, the valuable roles of other health professionals are now recognised and their input is formally encouraged. Patients are now managed in a multidisciplinary team whereby each member can share their skills, knowledge and expertise, for the patient's overall benefit.

Communicating with allied healthcare professionals

It is important when dealing with other healthcare professionals that you treat them with respect and dignity, and value their opinions. As members of the same team working for the patient's benefit, it is necessary to communicate well with one another and work in collaboration.

Teamwork

Working together and communicating between the various facets and disciplines is an essential component of teamwork. Ignoring the assessments and advice of other health professionals may adversely affect patient care. Imagine discharging a frail 89-year-old woman, who had been treated successfully with antibiotics for a UTI, without considering the physiotherapy or occupational therapy assessments regarding their mobility and home circumstances. Whilst the patient may be *medically* fit for discharge, other factors such as an inability to cope or mobilise could result in her speedy readmission.

Teams work more efficiently when they have a clear purpose, good communication and strong leadership. Whilst teams will be successful only if each and every member actively participates and is listened to, a recognised lead should be appointed to take the ultimate responsibility in the decision-making process. This position is often left to the Consultant, whose care the patient has ultimately been admitted under.

Respect

Doctors are trained to have a very good understanding about a wide range of diseases and disorders. Other healthcare professionals usually train for a similar period of time in their own particular disciplines. This means that they are likely to have a deeper understanding of certain issues relating to their speciality than a junior doctor would have. Hence, when their opinion is sought, it is important to value it, take it on board and act upon it. Being arrogant and dismissive of their opinions is non-conducive to the patient's well-being and is likely to unbalance the harmony of the team. Consider the following example:

Doctor: 'What seems to be concerning you about Mrs Jones's care?'

Stoma Nurse: 'Well, have you seen the way the stoma has been made? It's going to be an absolute nightmare for her to deal with!'

Doctor: 'She seems to be doing quite well otherwise. Considering the state she was in prior to her operation, she has made quite a remarkable recovery. The Consultant was saying that we could potentially send her home today?'

Stoma Nurse: 'I don't think that is a good idea.'

Doctor: 'What are your concerns? Perhaps I can relay them back to the Consultant.'

Stoma Nurse: 'She hasn't got to grips with her bag changes at all, and to be quite honest I don't think she ever will.'

Doctor: 'Hmmm . . . that is a difficulty. It's a shame given the fact that she is recovering so well otherwise. What do you suggest?'

Stoma Nurse: 'Well, I'll probably have to have a chat with one of the girls in the community and see whether they can do bag changes for her, but it might take me a while to sort that package out.'

In the above scenario, it would have been very easy for the doctor to dismiss the specialist nurse's opinion early on by stating that the Consultant had ordered the discharge. This may have resulted in the patient being prematurely discharged and would have caused a rebound admission due to stoma problems. However, the doctor managed to elicit the nurse's concerns and work with her to resolve any potential issues.

Communication

The multidisciplinary approach to healthcare requires all members of the team to work in tandem. This can only be effective if relevant information is correctly communicated between members. At times, the number of different disciplines involved in a patient's care may be quite large. It may be physically impossible to meet with and discuss all aspects of care with one another on a frequent basis. Clear, legible and well-documented notes recorded in a single file will permit the flow of information between the different specialities. In addition, having weekly MDT (multidisciplinary team) meetings, if feasible, will also help ensure that valuable assessments are discussed, considered and implemented.

The consultation: inter-professional communication

The way in which you introduce yourself to a colleague will be quite different to the way in which you do so to a patient. Usually with patients, your introduction will be more formal, whereas with colleagues it is often laid back and more casual.

The formalities of your introduction will vary depending on how well you know your colleague. A nurse with whom you work on a daily basis will probably not require much of an introduction. However, a dietician whom you will be meeting for the first time will probably need a more complete introduction, which should include your name and designation.

Following on from the introduction, the next step would be to try to establish rapport. Although there is an element of friendly 'banter' between colleagues, it is still important for the doctor to maintain an element of professionalism. Crossing the boundary may affect team spirit in the long run.

Establishing the problem

You may find yourself in a situation whereby you have requested a health professional to carry out a specific task *vis-à-vis* a patient, but it has not been performed and you are interested to find out why. Do not go charging in demanding answers as this is likely to lead to a confrontation and may not resolve the underlying problem. It is more conducive to simply ask your colleague the reasons for their perceived lack of action. In so doing you will be able to determine if they had understood the initial request or whether there were other mitigating circumstances preventing them from fulfilling it. Consider the following example:

Doctor:	'So, Joanne, why hasn't that child with appendicitis gone home yet? I completed the discharge form in good time and the Consultant expected him to be out of the door!'
Nurse:	'I am sorry but something came up!'
Doctor:	'That is unacceptable. The Consultant discharged the patient yesterday and all the forms have been completed. So, this begs the question, what caused the delay?'
Nurse:	'Yes . . . but . . .'
Doctor:	'I am sorry, but this child is occupying a bed for no reason. I hope it never happens again!'
Nurse:	'Fine!'

It is better to start off any discussion by gathering your colleague's understanding about the clinical situation. Give them ample opportunity to offer their opinion first, and show that you have acknowledged their explanation. It may be that they have a legitimate clinical reason for their action.

Doctor:	'So, Joanne, out of interest, why is that child with appendicitis still on the ward? Is anything the matter?'
Nurse:	'What, bed 17?'
Doctor:	'I thought I did his discharge form yesterday afternoon?'
Nurse:	'Yes, you did. But, something came up!'
Doctor:	'OK? What exactly happened?'
Nurse:	'There was something wrong with his medication.'
Doctor:	'Did I write his medications incorrectly?'
Nurse:	'No, no. Nothing like that. Yesterday we were seriously understaffed and I couldn't get the discharge form to Pharmacy in time before it closed.'
Doctor:	'I did not know that you were understaffed. I hope things are better today.'
Nurse:	'A little. But I have made it my priority to sort it out and the patient will be going home later on today.'

Acknowledging their reasons

Having spoken to your colleague about a particular concern you have, they may present you with a number of reasons as to why your request was not fulfilled. Try not to be dismissive of their excuses since their explanation may be genuine. You should acknowledge the difficulties they may have faced and show empathy if appropriate. This should enhance their trust and confidence in you and help you develop a suitable plan of action.

Discuss a plan

Hopefully by now you would have established good rapport with your colleague and gained an understanding of the problem at hand. Despite this, the fact remains that an important request was missed or delayed and the patient's care may have suffered as a result. It is your duty, therefore, to attempt to negotiate with your colleague an agreed management plan whereby the task can be completed. This undertaking may be more difficult than it first appears, particularly when the two parties are in disagreement. In such situations it is very important to take your colleague's point of view on board – after all they are part of the healthcare team and have expertise in areas that you do not have.

When there is a difference of opinion, try to understand why your colleague feels the way they do, and then put your point across. By showing them that you have taken their opinion seriously, it may be possible to come to common terms with them and find some middle ground.

Pharmacy: 'Doctor, I have some queries with regards to this discharge form. You've prescribed the patient Lansoprazole. I'm afraid in this Trust, we only use Omeprazole . . .'

Doctor: 'Hmm . . . my Consultant prefers using Lansoprazole and insists all his patients with reflux have it.'

Pharmacy: 'Yes, but it is Trust policy that our PPI of choice is Omeprazole. It is cheaper, and that's what the Chief Pharmacist has decided in conjunction with the hospital management.'

Doctor: 'Yes, but I think this particular patient is actually more suited to Lansoprazole. This patient prefers it as he used to be on Omeprazole, but his symptoms weren't controlled.'

Pharmacy: 'Well, I can't authorise this discharge form . . .'

Doctor: 'I appreciate where you are coming from. Although Trust guidelines are in place, they can change depending on the clinical situation. How about I discuss this with my Consultant first, and then we can take things from there?'

Pharmacy: 'Yes, I think that would be the most sensible thing to do . . .'

Inter-professional communication

The above framework should give you some understanding of how to tackle inter-professional communication. However, you will come into contact with a wide range of allied healthcare staff, with some of whom you will be on first name basis, and others who will be known to you more formally. In this section we will touch upon the roles of some of these staff members and useful ways of communicating with them.

Communicating with a nurse

Ward nurses are probably the most recognisable yet underappreciated staff members of the healthcare team. They are a common sight on any ward and represent the 'cogwheels' of the hospital. They are responsible for putting into motion doctors' requests for giving medication and charting patients' vital observations. Often if a patient is feeling unwell they will be the first person to know.

It is worth making yourself familiar with the various grades of nurses. Senior nurses are very experienced and are often in charge of the overall care of the ward. Junior nurses will usually be tasked with checking observations and are ultimately accountable to their charge nurses.

Communicating with a nurse specialist

In recent times, a new grade of nurse specialist has been introduced to the ward. You may have chanced upon them in the roles of diabetes nurse, pain nurse, heart failure nurse or even nurse endoscopists. These specialist nurses often hold their own outpatient clinics, provide advice on Consultant ward rounds and are even allowed to alter patient treatment within strict hospital protocols. They are quite experienced in their speciality and it is certainly worth taking their advice on board. However, if there is any disagreement in patient management you should always consult a senior member of your medical team.

Diabetes Nurse: 'Doctor, I was wondering if I could have a word with you about this prescription.'

Doctor: 'Sure, is there a problem?'

Diabetes Nurse: 'Whoever has prescribed this insulin regime clearly isn't familiar with the protocol. I've written about this in the notes, and I'm going to make the appropriate changes.'

Doctor: 'Well, it was actually the Registrar who made the management decision this morning, and he spoke to the Consultant about it after the ward round.'

Diabetes Nurse: 'But this goes against the hospital protocol I'm afraid. Let me show you the guidelines.' *(Shows them to Doctor)*

Doctor: *(After reading them)* 'Thank you for showing me this. I can understand your point of view, but sometimes, the Consultant chooses to deviate from protocols if they feel that the clinical situation indicates that they should do so. I think I'll have a chat with the Consultant about this patient, and discuss what you have told me before we make the changes. Is that OK?'

Diabetes Nurse: 'Yes, that's fine . . .'

Communicating with other healthcare professionals

There are numerous other disciplines that may be involved in the assessment and management of your patients. Your encounters with them may depend on the type of patient you are treating. If you are working in Care of the Elderly then you will frequently meet physiotherapists, occupational therapists, and speech and language therapists. Most of these therapists have trained in their given specialities for a number of years and may be quite experienced in their field. They often have a clearly defined role and when their opinion is sought their advice is highly regarded.

Communicating with the pharmacist

With regards to medications and their properties, pharmacists can offer a wealth of knowledge to doctors. For this reason, doctors and pharmacists typically have strong relationships. In some hospitals, pharmacists join the doctors' ward round, and are frequently called upon for their advice with regard to the most suitable drug for treating the patient. If the pharmacist offers you a drug which is perhaps more suited to the patient, it is certainly worth considering. However, if there is any uncertainty about their advice, then you should consult with your senior, as the ultimate responsibility for prescribing lies with the doctors. Pharmacists are often acutely aware of drug formularies, costings and local hospital drug protocols, which newly inducted doctors, may not have much knowledge about.

Communicating with administrative staff

There are many members of staff who work behind the scenes to ensure that patients receive the care they need, such as outpatient follow-ups, referrals to other hospitals and operations. It is important for the doctor to remember that these staff may not necessarily be medically qualified. Therefore, when communicating with them, complex medical jargon needs to be avoided.

Communicating about a clinical incident

A particularly demanding aspect of inter-professional communication is talking to another team member about a clinical incident which they were directly involved in. The challenge in such a scenario is to highlight the error to the person involved without causing offence or attributing blame.

When a clinical incident has taken place, it is important not to speak to the person involved in an aggressive tone, nor humiliate them in front of other team members. None of us ever intend to make a mistake, and we have all been in situations of intense stress which have caused us to fall into error. Thus, before discussing a clinical incident with a colleague, you should try to put yourself in their position and consider whether there could be a simple explanation as to why things went wrong.

Try to familiarise yourself with the nature of the clinical incident before approaching your colleague. It is good practice to take time out to read the clinical and nursing notes together, to establish a clear picture of what took place at the time of the incident, and where and why errors may have occurred.

When dealing with situations of potential conflict, the communication skills needed are similar to those of breaking bad news. To avoid feelings of shock and annoyance, give details in small bite-sized chunks. Always remember to explore how it makes them feel and check understanding before moving on. Consider the example below:

Doctor:	'Lisa, we had a meeting to discuss the care of Mr James, and it emerged that there were aspects of his care that were suboptimal. The Consultant asked me to investigate this matter as a clinical incident so that we can learn from it and hopefully prevent it from happening again.'
Lisa:	'Really? Is there is anything I could do to help?'
Doctor:	'Well, after examining his notes, we found that he had been without IV fluids for almost 12 hours in the immediate post-operative period and this was the main reason as to why he developed acute renal failure.'
Lisa:	'OK . . .'
Doctor:	'According to the notes you were the nurse in charge of his bay during this period. The IV fluids had been written up by the doctor but unfortunately they were not administered. Do you remember what happened on that day?'
Lisa:	'I can vaguely remember that day. We were short staffed and had three crash calls on the ward. It must have slipped my mind with all the commotion.'
Doctor:	'Lisa, I fully understand your difficulties. I know what it's like to be short staffed. However, for the patient's benefit we want to put guidelines in place to prevent this from happening again. It may be an idea to put forward any ideas or proposals that we could consider in the meeting tomorrow?'

Lisa: 'Oh, that's a good idea. I'll think about the matter tonight and have a discussion with the rest of the nurses and we will see what we can come up with for tomorrow.'

FIRST CLINICAL SCENARIO

Premature patient discharge

Communicating with allied healthcare professionals is a vital skill that a doctor is required to be accomplished in. A breakdown in communication can have serious consequences to patient care and management. It is important to be empathic and allow your colleague enough time to explain possible reasons why things did not go as planned. Do not try to be blameworthy. Instead, encourage all those involved to learn from the mistake so as to reduce the possibility of its reoccurrence.

DOCTOR'S BRIEF

You are the Care of the Elderly ST2. You have recently been looking after Mr Ramsey, a 78-year-old man who was admitted following a chest infection. He has completed his course of intravenous antibiotics and is medically fit for discharge. You decide after today's ward round that he can go home. Whilst in the doctors' mess, the ward sister bleeps you saying the physiotherapist wants to have a word about Mr Ramsey's care.

ACTOR'S BRIEF *(if you are the doctor, please do not read)*

You are a Physiotherapist, and you have just been informed that one of your patients, Mr Ramsey, has been deemed to be medically fit for discharge. You are quite annoyed by this decision as in your opinion the patient is not fit for discharge and you have communicated this clearly in the patient's notes. You are feeling very frustrated, as you feel as if the team are ignoring all the hard work you are putting in trying to mobilise the patient. You have informed the ward sister that you would like to speak to the doctor looking after Mr Ramsey.

SCENARIO WALK-THROUGH

INTRODUCE YOURSELF	*Doctor:*	'Hello. My name is Dr Gregory. I'm one of the doctors looking after Mr Ramsey. I'm relatively new on the ward and I don't think we have met.'
	Physio:	*'My name is Hugh and I'm the physio for the ward. I'm glad you've taken the time out to see me.'*
ESTABLISH COLLEAGUE'S IDEAS	*Doctor:*	'Well, the sister in charge told me you wanted to have a word about Mr Ramsey.'
	Physio:	*'Well yes! And to be quite honest, I'm sick and tired of your team making decisions without consulting anyone else . . .'*
ELICIT COLLEAGUE'S CONCERNS	*Doctor:*	'What seems to be concerning you, Hugh?'
ALLOW YOUR COLLEAGUE TO VENT THEIR ANGER	*Physio:*	*'You doctors need to understand that it's not just you guys who care for the patient. We're all here to help! Now, Mr Ramsey came in with a chest infection, and he's been in for a while!*
		'Just because you've treated his chest infection doesn't mean he can go home straight away! Do you even read the physiotherapy notes?
	PAUSE	
		'Do you know that he is still having difficulty going up and down the stairs, which he could do before he was admitted? His legs have become more weak whilst he has been here, but you've probably not even bothered to check, or even asked anyone! I am absolutely astounded that you have written in the notes "Home today". There is no way he can go home!'
DEMONSTRATE UNDERSTANDING AND SHOW EMPATHY	*Doctor:*	'I am sorry you feel this way, Hugh. You are quite right. When we treat our patients we usually try to take into account all those who are involved with their care, including, of course, physiotherapists. However, in this case we were not made aware that there was an issue with his mobility.'
	Physio:	*'It is quite clear you haven't even bothered to read what I wrote!'*
	Doctor:	'Well, I think part of the difficulty lies in the fact that there are separate sections in the medical notes for

		the physiotherapist, which are often quite hard to locate quickly.'
	Physio:	'That is true. But still, that doesn't stop you from asking one of us about how a patient is doing from our perspective. You know, it really makes me feel worthless when you guys just go ahead and make a decision on discharge when we are still treating a patient.'
EMPATHISE	Doctor:	'Once again I do apologise, and you certainly are not worthless members of the team. Were it not for the hard work you put into patient mobility, many of our patients wouldn't leave hospital, and we certainly appreciate that. Why don't we address your concerns with regard to Mr Ramsey's care first and foremost, and perhaps we can later think of ways of improving communication between our teams?'
	Physio:	'Going back to Mr Ramsey. As I said, before, he was able to manage going up and down stairs. He's lost a lot of confidence whilst being in hospital, and we're trying to build that back up again. If we sent him now, he'd probably pitch up again in A&E as the result of a fall!'
ASK OPINION, GIVE THEM IMPORTANCE	Doctor:	'Right – do you think you can get him back up to speed?'
	Physio:	'No, not to how he originally was. I was wondering whether it would be worth having an OT assess his house to see if there is anything they can offer?'
	Doctor:	'Do you think that would be useful to you?'
	Physio:	'Well, it's not worth us just discharging him, and then him returning back to hospital due to an accident in the home. Whilst he was quite capable of managing his daily tasks before coming in, I still think an assessment would be useful . . .'
IN A HEATED SITUATION, DEFEND YOURSELF WHEN APPROPRIATE	Doctor:	'I can see your point of view. However, it can sometimes be difficult to appreciate each and every aspect of the patient care on our ward rounds. With time constraints it is difficult for us to keep abreast of the social issues alongside their medical ones.'

Physio:		*'I understand, Doctor. It's just quite frustrating sometimes.'*
Doctor:		'So, when do you anticipate that Mr Ramsey will be ready for discharge, so that we both can have a date to work towards?'
Physio:		*'I think he should be close to his maximum potential in about five days from now, and I think that that should be enough time to organise an OT assessment.'*
ELICIT LONGSTANDING CONCERNS	*Doctor:*	'Good, I'm glad that is cleared up. Now I understand that you were angry, and it seems as if this frustration has been building up for a while now ...'
	Physio:	*'Thanks for that. But it still doesn't solve the problem of miscommunication between our teams.'*
OFFER SOLUTION	*Doctor:*	'OK, how about if you joined our ward round once a week, to update us on the progress of some of the patients?'
	Physio:	*'I think that may be useful for us but we also rely on OT, social services and dieticians.'*
	Doctor:	'OK. It would make sense if we could all meet up at a specific time during the week on a regular basis, like in an MDT meeting?'
	Physio:	*'I think that is a very good idea. I'll take it back to the other therapists and see what we can do about it.'*
	Doctor:	'Fine. I will also get back to my team and get back to you by next week. It sounds promising.'
	Physio:	*'OK. I'll see you then.'*

CONSULTATION ENDS

Delayed analgesia given to a patient

Communicating directives with allied healthcare professionals is part of a doctor's daily routine. If such communication breaks down, essential medical care for the patient may be overlooked. On occasions this may be serious enough to reach the level of a clinical incident. How you go about discussing these sensitive issues with your colleagues may make or break inter-professional relationships.

DOCTOR'S BRIEF

You are the Surgical ST2. You have decided to come to work a little early as you wish to review your patients before the morning handover meeting. You go to see Mr Naylor who recently had a procedure. He complains to you that he asked the nurse to give him some analgesia overnight, and that he had to wait four hours before it was administered. He was also upset with the nurse's attitude and behaviour towards him when confronted. He is threatening to lodge a formal complaint with the hospital. To calm the patient you have agreed to discuss the incident with the nurse involved.

ACTOR'S BRIEF *(if you are the doctor, please do not read)*

You are Julie Brown, a staff nurse. You have just been working the night shift, and it has been incredibly stressful for you, as you had to deal with two back-to-back crash calls. In addition, one of the patients, Mr Naylor, was constantly ringing the bell last night with what seemed to be trivial requests. You do recall however, that he did ask for some analgesia, but due to crash calls, there was a long delay before you gave it to him. The patient was left frustrated and not receptive to your reasons. Generally, you are quite passionate about your job, but you also don't take any nonsense from anybody!

SCENARIO WALK-THROUGH

INTRODUCE YOURSELF	*Doctor:*	'Hi, Julie, how's it going?'
	Nurse:	*'Not too bad, Doctor, and yourself?'*
ESTABLISH RAPPORT	*Doctor:*	'Everything is fine. Nice and fresh for the morning! How did your shift go?'
	Nurse:	*'Oh, it was a real nightmare. We had two crash calls overnight, you know!'*
	Doctor:	'Oh really?'
	Nurse:	*'Yeah, two of the post-ops arrested. I really wish the day teams would review their patients more often! They were showing signs of going off during the day and it seems nobody even batted an eyelid!'*
TRY TO OFFER A SOLUTION TO THE CONCERN	*Doctor:*	'OK, I'll be going to the morning handover shortly, and I'm sure we'll be discussing it there. I'll raise your concerns with the team in charge of those patients.'
	Nurse:	*'Yes, please do . . .'*
PRIVACY	*Doctor:*	'Julie, there is something that I wanted to talk to you about. Is it OK if we go to the office?'
	Nurse:	*'Is everything OK?'*
	Doctor:	'Yes, nothing to be alarmed about; I just needed some clarification that's all . . .'

ENTER OFFICE

	Doctor:	'Well, Julie, it's about Mr Naylor . . .'
	Nurse:	*'Oh yeah! Mr Naylor . . .' (Says sarcastically)*
OPEN QUESTION, ESTABLISH COLLEAGUE'S IDEAS	*Doctor:*	'Why do you say that?'
	Nurse:	*'Doctor, he has got to be the most impatient person I have ever met! He's always ringing the bell asking for something! Honestly, when there are a million and one things to do, it can really get on your nerves!'*
DEMONSTRATE UNDERSTANDING AND SHOW EMPATHY	*Doctor:*	'Ah yes, it can get a little difficult at times . . .'
	Nurse:	*'Huh, a little!'*
	Doctor:	'I appreciate that you had a particularly busy night with some rather sick patients, and that Mr Naylor may have added to the aggravation. But I just went to check up on him before handover this morning, and he wasn't too pleased.'
	Nurse:	*'Now why doesn't that surprise me?!'*

ESTABLISH COLLEAGUE'S PERSPECTIVE	*Doctor:*	'Do you know of anything in particular that could have made him so upset?'
	Nurse:	*'Well, he did ask for some analgesia in the middle of the night, and I went to draw it up. Then both crash calls happened straight after one another, and it was about four hours after that, before I actually gave it to him. Then he had a go at me on the ward in front of all the patients!'*
	Doctor:	'That sounds quite unfortunate . . . Obviously I can see where you are coming from. Crash calls are quite stressful, and he was probably quite agitated at not being given his analgesia, resulting in the argument.'
	Nurse:	*'I'm not superwoman you know!'*
ELICIT COLLEAGUE'S CONCERNS	*Doctor:*	'The thing is, Julie, he is threatening to lodge a formal complaint.'
	Nurse:	*'The cheek . . . I work so hard, and that's the repayment I get . . .'*
EXPECTATIONS – OFFER A POTENTIAL SOLUTION	*Doctor:*	'I can totally agree that last night must have been very rushed. For Mr Naylor – he was post-op and in considerable pain which can also be quite frustrating. I think there might have been a simple breakdown in communication, and I think that just by explaining the situation to him, we can avoid a formal complaint.'
	Nurse:	*'Look Doctor, he drives me up the wall, I'm not going to see him again. I'm tired and I wanna go home.'*
NEGOTIATE	*Doctor:*	'How about if we both go to him? We can explain the difficulties you had last night, and apologise that he had to wait so long, but that there was a valid reason for it. You know, just saying that much can sometimes have a profound effect and prevent the stress of a formal complaint.'
	Nurse:	*'Hmmm . . . OK . . . I guess you are right. It would make things much easier tonight too, because I'm on again . . .!'*
	Doctor:	'Excellent. I'm sure we can resolve this amicably.'

CONSULTATION ENDS

CHAPTER 9

Apologising for mistakes

Mistakes are part and parcel of human nature and everyone is prone to making them. They can range from being simple or benign to the catastrophic or terminal. Although society tends to portray doctors as being 'all-knowing' and 'infallible', doctors, like any other profession, are just as likely to make mistakes and fall into error.

Unfortunately, mistakes will happen, but although they are demoralising, learning from mistakes and taking steps to rectify them is as important as avoiding them in the first place. As doctors, although we may find it hard to accept that we have fallen into error, this should not prevent us from seeking advice, improving on our knowledge and being open and honest as to what has occurred.

Mistakes

In medicine, mistakes take place on a daily basis. They range from simple clerical errors of spelling to the removal of the wrong kidney. Studies have shown that in the UK around one in ten patients suffer an adverse event during their time in hospital. Given the huge number of patients the NHS sees on a yearly basis this is a worryingly high figure. Whilst mistakes are inevitable, how one goes about dealing with the consequences will have a strong bearing on the outcome.

Whilst it may seem easy to try to conceal a mistake in the hope that it will not be discovered, this runs contrary to the professional standards of a doctor and is wholly irresponsible and dishonest.

Probity

Probity as defined by the GMC is being 'honest and trustworthy, acting with integrity'. This is the heart of medical professionalism and maintains the public's trust in us. One should never allow this key principle to be compromised, as this may bring yourself or the profession into disrepute.

In the context of making mistakes, it is expected that you would declare any failings to your patient, and if relevant, to your peers or professional body.

Although it may be difficult to admit to *yourself* that you have erred, especially when the mistake may have far-reaching consequences on your career and status, it takes even more courage to admit it to *others*. More often than not, by being brave and honest one gains the respect and trust of the patient, as well as your fellow professionals. On the other hand, if you were found to have concealed your mistake, you may be open to litigation and expulsion from the profession by the GMC.

Documentation

Patient notes are legal documents that record a timeline of care provided to the patient. They are usually open to a variety of medical and allied professionals to write in. When documenting in the notes, you should clearly state the date and time of your entry and sign and write your name. Although it may seem obvious, take care that all your entries are fully legible, as scruffy and illegible notes may be interpreted as a lack of care and due concern. It is very difficult to prove that you performed a particular task at a given time if you cannot back your claim up with documented evidence. The basic principle holds that 'if it is not recorded in the notes, it did not take place'. You should never alter or amend previous entries in the notes even if what you document is true, as this may be interpreted as a deceitful attempt to change the facts.

When mistakes happen

Mistakes are rarely restricted to the fault of a single individual. They usually occur due to failure in systems, protocols or as a result of unforeseen events. For this reason, if you believe a mistake has been committed it is good practice to flag your concern to a senior colleague on your firm. It may be useful to sit down with this person and discuss the clinical case in depth. Your colleague may be able to help you identify what went wrong, establish who is potentially responsible and suggest ways to discuss this with the patient. They may also be able to provide constructive advice as to how to avoid repeating the same mistake again and what lessons can be learnt.

Medical indemnity

All doctors and hospital trusts are obliged to have medical indemnity insurance. Apart from providing assistance in litigious matters they also provide advisory services when mistakes happen. Depending on the magnitude of the mistake it may be advisable to contact your indemnity provider to clarify the next best course of action.

Clinical incident form

When mistakes occur, one should complete a clinical incident form. The term 'clinical incident' is an umbrella term used to describe events which have or had the potential to cause unintentional physical or mental harm. An 'adverse event' is one in which such harm has taken place, whereas 'near miss' describes an event where no harm has occurred but could easily have done so.

Clinical incident form reporting is regarded as an essential tool in maintaining patient safety. The reporting of such events enables areas of concern to be highlighted and appraised so as to improve the quality of patient care and safety, in a blame-free manner.

The clinical incident form should be filled out early and without delay. You should try to record the events that led up to the mistake as you remember them. You should also highlight areas that you felt had gone wrong and what you did to try to rectify them. Make sure local protocols regarding clinical incidents are adhered to and the form is sent to the relevant departments as soon as possible.

The consultation

Regardless of magnitude or impact on the patient, all mistakes should be acknowledged and the patient informed. Accepting that one has made a mistake and admitting it to the patient, may seem like a mammoth task. However, with careful preparation and planning one may be able undertake this task successfully, minimising complaints and any subsequent fallout.

Preparation

Once you realise you have made a mistake, the first thing to do is to acknowledge it. You need to be honest enough to admit it to yourself and to your colleagues. The patient always has a right to know and it is better to explain things now rather than keeping them in the dark. You should, therefore, mentally prepare yourself to discuss things with the patient and/or their relatives.

Patient's notes

It is important to obtain access to the full set of the patient's notes to try to establish when the mistake took place. Reading through the notes will also help you to catalogue the events that led up to the mistake, revealing any failings of protocols or procedure. It will also help you to be fully aware of the facts prior to your discussion with the patient.

on their rounds. Mind you, I reckon I'd be quite upset if it was true!'

Explaining the mistake

It may be apparent that the patient is aware that something has gone wrong and will require a frank explanation with regards to this. If the patient is not aware that a mistake has taken place, now would be an ideal time to inform them. You should use clear, unambiguous language when explaining what has happened. It may be useful to start with the phrase *'I'm afraid we've made a slight error'*, or *'I'm afraid that things did not entirely go as planned'*. Do not forget to allow for pauses, before going on to explain the nature of the mistake. This will allow the patent time to digest and appreciate what they have just been told.

Doctor:	'Well. It is true that you were given a different drug to what you normally take. *PAUSE* 'Unfortunately, an error was made on your drug chart . . .'
Mr Simon:	'I see . . .'
Doctor:	'I inadvertently wrote another patient's drug on your chart, and it was given to you this morning before I could correct it . . .'

Make an apology

Very often, a simple apology is all it takes to solve a patient's grievance. Unfortunately, medical professionals often hesitate in performing this simple task early on as it is perceived as an admission of guilt. More often than not, you will be worried about how the mistake reflects back on your reputation, or that the patient has an unforgiving persona and may take things further. The key thing to remember is that an apology does not necessarily equate to an admission of guilt.

It is important that you are careful when you apologise to the patient. In situations where you are apologising on behalf of others, you may appear to be taking personal blame for the mistake. In such circumstances it is better to use terms such as *'we'* and *'us'* to refer to the team as a whole. Consider the following example, where a doctor is apologising for a mistake his colleague made:

Patient:	'Hi, Doctor. Have you come to take me to theatre? I've been waiting since morning for this operation and I was told that it should have happened already!'
Doctor:	'I'm really sorry for the delay. But we have had to cancel the operation as you have just eaten.'

Patient:	'What! I hadn't eaten since morning, but an hour ago one of your nurses brought me up some food and said I could eat.'
Doctor:	'I am sorry. I feel really bad for you.'
Patient:	'There's no good feeling bad about it! You're supposed to be a professional and know what you're doing! You guys gave me the food and now my operation is cancelled.'
Doctor:	'I know. I'm so sorry. I wish this didn't happen. I'm sorry.'

Anyone listening to the conversation would assume that it was the doctor himself who made the error. The doctor, by apologising in the way he has, appears to have taken all the blame for the mistake, making him appear incompetent in the eyes of the patient. Instead of advising the patient of what steps can be taken to rectify the problem, the doctor has preoccupied himself solely with apologising. In so doing, this may cause the patient to lose their trust in the doctor's ability and subsequent performance in conducting the operation.

The following example illustrates how this situation may have been handled better:

Patient:	'You guys gave me the food and now my operation is cancelled!'
Doctor:	'Yes. I'd like to offer a full apology on behalf of the team, that this mistake has happened. However, we have taken steps to rectify this by rebooking you to have the operation in six hours' time. I have also written a clear sign on your chart that you should not be allowed to eat anything before the operation.'
Patient:	'Well . . . I guess mistakes can happen, and I can see you're trying to sort it out.'

Things to avoid when apologising

When apologising to the patient you should not shift the blame of the mistake on to others or attempt to conceal your mistake. You should also avoid being evasive or adopting a confrontational manner when responding to questions. This will inevitably lead to problems during your consultation and make your apology appear half-hearted.

Attaching blame

Be careful of falling into the trap of blaming yourself or anyone else for the mistake. Apologising for a mistake, or acknowledging that one has been made, does not mean that you are 'owning up' or accepting culpability.

Apportioning blame for a particular mistake will often detract from the main matter of rectifying the problem and may cause mistrust between colleagues. Creating a blame-free environment is more likely to facilitate people to own up to their individual mistakes. This will allow systems to be put into place to rectify problems and prevent reoccurrence.

Consider the following example of a House Officer explaining a prescribing error that his Consultant made on the ward round:

Patient:	'I cannot believe that I was given the wrong injection! Don't you doctors know what you are doing? How long have you been qualified?'
Doctor:	'I am very sorry for this mistake, Mr Wilson. I have rectified the error and have filled out an incident form, which means that this will be investigated fully.'
Patient:	'Didn't you learn anything at medical school? Why didn't you speak to the Consultant before you gave it to me?'
Doctor:	'Well . . . in fact it was the Consultant who made the mistake and told me to prescribe it!'
Patient:	'Well . . . Why didn't YOU check it?'

This exchange, which has culminated in the blame being directed at the Consultant has completely shifted the emphasis from learning from mistakes to finger pointing. This is likely to damage the relationship the patient has with the individual and the wider team, as well as create dissent within the team itself. In the example above, the Consultant may also be likely to face further difficulties when he next meets the patient during a ward round and in future consultations. Now consider how this could have been handled in a different way:

Patient:	'I cannot believe that I was given the wrong injection! Don't you doctors know what you are doing? How long have you been qualified?'
Doctor:	'I am very sorry for this mistake, Mr Wilson. I have rectified the error and have filled out an incident form, which means that this will be investigated fully.'
Patient:	'Didn't you learn anything at medical school? Why didn't you speak to the Consultant before you gave it to me?'
Doctor:	'I can only apologise again for the mistake. I can assure you that we take these matters very seriously and we will be investigating how the mistake occurred. We have already put into place procedures that will help prevent it from happening again. From now onwards we will be cross-checking the drug chart with the details on your

wristband as well as the information in your notes, before prescribing.'

Patient: 'OK then . . . as long as it does not happen again . . .'

In the second example the doctor has apologised for the mistake on behalf of the team. In his response to the patient he has clearly focused on highlighting the lessons that had been learnt and the processes that have been implemented to prevent similar mistakes from happening in the future. By doing this, the patient's confidence in health professionals should remain intact and their trust in the health service remains unscathed.

Confrontation

When informing a patient or relative that a mistake has happened, there is a risk that the encounter may turn confrontational. The patient may be left surprised and shocked that a mistake had taken place. They may wish to confront you in order to gain more information as to how and why it occurred. The doctor may fuel the patient's frustration by evading their line of questioning (in order to avoid blame) or by providing contradictory statements. Consider the following example:

Doctor: 'Hello. I'm Dr Anderson. Are you Mrs Rhodes's daughter?'

Daughter: 'Yes. I am pleased to meet you.'

Doctor: 'I understand that you are unhappy at something that has happened during your mother's stay. Is that right?'

Daughter: 'Well, I'm not happy that she seems to be losing weight since she has been in hospital.'

Doctor: 'I see. You are obviously quite concerned by this.'

Daughter: 'Yes, I am. Every time she comes to hospital you pump her full of drugs that stop her from eating. When she is at home with me she is completely fine.'

Doctor: 'The drugs we are giving her help with her blood pressure and her diabetes which are important for her health.'

Daughter: 'No . . . Can't you see you are harming her!'

Doctor: 'Sorry! I don't understand. I do not accept your claim that I am intentionally harming your mother.'

Daughter: 'Yes . . . no. I mean don't get me wrong, not directly . . .'

Doctor: 'I think I have heard enough. I will not accept your accusations and I cannot continue with this conversation.'

Daughter: 'Hold it right there . . . Don't you walk away!'

In the example above, the doctor had intended to meet with the patient's relative to discuss an issue of concern with her. Unfortunately, due to miscommunication and a confrontational approach, the meeting almost descended into a slanging match of blame and counter blame. The doctor felt that the patient's relative was insinuating that they were intentionally seeking to harm her mother, although this was clearly not the case. Instead of exploring the relative's worries and concerns in more depth, the doctor has taken the statements at face value and reacted accordingly. By avoiding a confrontational approach, it is likely the above disagreement could have been circumvented.

As a general rule, you should avoid direct confrontation with the patient or their relatives as much as possible. In a case where the patient or their relative becomes confrontational, you should attempt to ease things by remaining calm, using phrases which demonstrate empathy and encouraging the patient or their relative to express their feelings. Remember, it is more difficult to recover a consultation when both parties have lost their cool.

Evasiveness and covering up

When apologising to the patient it is important to be truthful, honest and open, regardless of what may have taken place. It is unbecoming of a health professional to be evade the patient's questions, especially if they are attempting to establish what went wrong. You should also never consider covering up your mistakes, as this is not in keeping with the characteristics of good medical practice. Consider the following example:

Patient: 'I'd like to say that I'm not very happy with my care. Apparently you've known I've had a wound infection for several days and yet only today did you start me on antibiotics. Is this true?'

Doctor: 'Well, Mr Fox, it depends on which way you look at it. You know most of us have got bugs on our skin and yet we don't all take antibiotics . . .'

Patient: 'I want to know if on this occasion I should have started taking antibiotics earlier or not?'

Doctor: 'Look Mr Fox, medicine is an art, not a science. These things are all about subtle judgements and vary from case to case so things can be delayed or done earlier. In your case that decision was a bit tricky.'

Patient: 'Who's responsible for the decision not to give me antibiotics?'

Doctor: 'Again Mr Fox, it is not as simple as that. We don't work as individuals in the hospital but rather work in teams adopting a multidisciplinary approach. When it comes to infections, we take guidance from the microbiologists.

Even though technically we make the final decision, it is unheard of not to follow their advice. But I must admit, your results were a little bit delayed because of the Bank Holiday weekend.'

Patient: 'So, it's the microbiologist's fault then?'

Doctor: 'Well, not exactly.'

As you can see, the doctor is avoiding giving any clear answers and is essentially refusing to acknowledge that an error has occurred. He is seemingly rambling on in the hope that he can avoid the very real issue of a possible mistake and its ramifications. Whilst he may have very noble intentions, this approach is ignoring the right of the patient to be kept fully informed about their care. For this reason, it is important to be honest with facts and recognise that mistakes have been made. This approach, in addition to being principled, will be appreciated by patients far more than one which is evasive and ambiguous.

Eliciting the patient's concerns

By now you would have informed the patient of the mistake and made a genuine attempt at an apology. If the patient was unaware of the error, it is highly likely that fresh worries may be developing in their mind. It is important for you to pick up on any verbal or non-verbal cues from the patient, such as changes in their demeanour or signs of worry in their facial expression, which may reveal to you the degree of anxiety that they harbour.

It is important that you try to address these concerns instead of allowing them to brew and ferment into a fully fledged complaint. Consider the following example:

Doctor: 'Mr Phillips, although you have told me you are happy with our plan following this unfortunate mistake, you seem a little troubled about something. Is there anything worrying you?'

Patient: 'Well, to be honest, Doctor, I'm just a bit worried about having a delayed reaction to the drug . . . when you are not around, like if I go to the toilet or in the middle of the night . . . I know you've said that I should be in the clear and you'll all keep an eye on me, but what will happen if something goes wrong when I'm on my own?'

Doctor: 'I appreciate your concerns. I just want to reassure you that if you should feel unwell at any time, you can pull the patient cord and someone will be with you straight away. I will make sure I hand things over to the night staff so that

	they regularly check on you and that you are doing fine. How does that sound?'
Patient:	'Thanks, Doctor, I feel reassured by that.'

Elicit the patient's expectations and explain the next steps

It is feasible that the patient, who is now aware of the mistake, has their own ideas about what should be done. Their trust and confidence in your ability may have been shaken and henceforward they may become more demanding as to what should happen next. The patient may make unreasonable requests and these should be dealt with sympathetically but firmly. Consider the following example:

Doctor:	'Now that we realise our mistake, we will keep a close eye on you for 24 hours and do a blood test tomorrow morning. As long as you remain well and the blood test is OK, we will let you go home after that. How does that sound to you?'
Patient:	'I'm sorry, but I'm still not happy with what has happened. I want to be absolutely sure that by your delaying my antibiotics, my chest infection has not worsened. I want an urgent CT scan to make sure this is not the case. You've made this mistake, and I want to make sure it is put right!'

Although it is clear from the example that the patient's demands are entirely unreasonable, it is important not to completely dismiss his demands as being absurd. Rather, you should try to reassure the patient that with observation and re-examination they will be fit for discharge and a routine chest X-ray will be repeated in due course.

Doctor:	'I appreciate your concerns and understand that you are not happy that the antibiotic had been missed. However, I would like to reassure you that, after performing a detailed examination, checking your most recent blood tests and monitoring your observations, we are confident that the missed antibiotic dose has not had any adverse effect upon you. We would like to keep you in hospital for another 24 hours to be absolutely certain that you are well enough for discharge.
	PAUSE
	'As you are well in yourself, we do not feel that a CT scan would change how we will be treating you and it would entail an unnecessary high dose of radiation. Your last chest

X-ray showed us that your chest infection is improving and we will be repeating this in six weeks' time when we will see you again in clinic to make sure it has completely resolved. Obviously, if anything changes in the meantime we will be more than happy to see you earlier.'

Explain how you will avoid this mistake again

Inform the patient that your organisation is committed to minimising risk to patients and maximising their safety, and, for this reason, you are filling out a clinical incident form. Explain that the purpose of this is so that the incident can be investigated fully and so that any lessons learnt can be acted upon.

If there are any other specific steps you are taking, for example holding meetings or having discussions with seniors, give brief details of these plans to the patient in order to demonstrate that you are being proactive in dealing with the problem. By doing this you will reassure the patient that you have taken their concerns seriously and that, hopefully, the mistake will never be repeated.

Summarising back and closing up

Before you close the meeting with the patient you should enquire as to whether they have any further questions or concerns that they would like to discuss with you. It is always a good idea to summarise back to the patient what you have discussed; this gives you the opportunity to check that they have understood everything that has been stated and jointly agree on the next course of action.

Doctor: 'Before we finish, I would just like to summarise some of the points we have discussed today. You were admitted two days ago with a chest infection. We had decided today to repeat your chest X-ray. Unfortunately, a member of our team requested an abdominal X-ray by mistake and this was the investigation that took place.
PAUSE
'We apologise unreservedly for this mistake and we have filed a clinical incident report in order to ensure that this incident is investigated appropriately and steps are taken to make sure it does not happen again.
PAUSE
'We have spoken to the X-ray department who have informed us that the risks to your health as a result of this mix up are extremely small. As a team, we have decided that we can minimise the risk of these mistakes occurring

	if we delegate a single member of staff to be responsible for checking all the requests. Are you happy with this?'
Patient:	'Yes, Doctor, thank you for sorting it all out. I really hope it will not happen again and I will see you in the morning.'

Housekeeping

It is quite easy to have your confidence shaken when a mistake has happened. Despite apologising to the patient, feelings of guilt may still persist within you. Consider taking a few minutes to collect your thoughts after the consultation. You may wish to discuss the case with a senior colleague or your own educational supervisor who may be able to offer you additional advice and support and help bring the matter to a close.

CLINICAL SCENARIO

Drug allergy

When a mistake has occurred and it has had, or may have had, an effect on the patient's well-being, it is appropriate that the patient is informed. The patient will more often than not find out this fact regardless of any attempt to conceal it. Deliberately attempting to cover up mistakes may raise questions regarding your fitness to practice and professional conduct.

DOCTOR'S BRIEF

You are a Foundation Year doctor in General Medicine. Henry Seeward is a 46-year-old man who was admitted yesterday evening with community-acquired pneumonia. He is stable and making a fast recovery. You happened to be the doctor who clerked him in yesterday and initiated his management with amoxicillin. During the post-take ward round, you notice a copy of the casualty card which you also had access to when you first saw the patient. In the allergies section it reads *'penicillin'*. However, you forgot to ask the patient at the time and did not notice it yesterday.

After realising your mistake, you make the necessary alterations to the drug chart, complete an incident form and call the microbiologist, who has informed you that you should change to an alternative antibiotic. He also advises you that it is unlikely that the patient has a severe drug allergy to penicillin, as they haven't yet developed a drug reaction despite having taken two doses. You have spoken to the charge nurse, who has advised you to discuss this mistake with the patient. The patient requests to see you to discuss why his medication has been changed.

ACTOR'S BRIEF *(if you are the doctor, please do not read)*

You are Henry Seeward, a 46-year-old man who was admitted yesterday evening with pneumonia. You are relieved that you received treatment in good time and are making a fast recovery. However, earlier today you noticed the doctor come in and make changes to your medication chart without informing you. You are concerned that you will now be receiving a weaker drug that will not be as effective. You are not aware that you have been given penicillin for the pneumonia as you did mention to the triage nurse that you were allergic to it. You recall your mother telling you that you once came out in a rash as a child after being given penicillin and have always remembered to mention your allergy when asked. You realise that doctors have a difficult and stressful job and that mistakes are made and you do not wish to make their job harder. However, what you cannot stand is being kept in the dark or not being given the full picture.

SCENARIO WALK-THROUGH

INTRODUCE YOURSELF TO THE PATIENT AND ESTABLISH RAPPORT	*Doctor:*	'Hello, Mr Seeward. I'm Dr Phillips. How are you today?'
	Mr S:	*'Yes, not bad, Doctor.'*
	Doctor:	'How have things been for you since you came into hospital?'
	Mr S:	*'Well, obviously I'm much better now. I was in a right state when I came in, but not doing so bad now, thanks.'*
ESTABLISH PURPOSE OF CONSULTATION	*Doctor:*	'I understand that you wanted to talk to a doctor about a particular concern you have had about your care. Is this correct?'
	Mr S:	*'Yes. That's right. I am a little concerned that my treatment had been changed recently.'*
ESTABLISH PATIENT'S CONCERNS	*Doctor:*	'Do you mind telling me more about what you are concerned about?'
	Mr S:	*'Well . . . I've got this pneumonia in my lungs, and I'm sure that I started getting better after the first dose of the antibiotic you gave me . . . I've had two doses of the stuff and now I've been told that you've changed it!'*
EXPLAIN MISTAKE	*Doctor:*	'I'm afraid we've made a mistake with one of your medications.'
	PAUSE	
	Mr S:	*'Mistake? What kind of mistake?'*
	Doctor:	'When you first came in we diagnosed you with pneumonia and started treatment with antibiotics. The first antibiotic we used was amoxicillin.'
	Mr S:	*'OK, so is that the antibiotic you stopped?'*
	Doctor:	'Yes, because it is a penicillin-containing antibiotic.'
	Mr S:	*'Penicillin! I'm allergic to penicillin!'*
APOLOGISE/EXPLAIN	*Doctor:*	'Yes. I am sorry that we overlooked that fact. It seems that a mistake occurred, but thankfully we have stopped the drug before any harm has taken place.'
	PAUSE	
	Mr S:	*'OH MY GOD!'*

Doctor: 'Fortunately you have not had any adverse reaction to it. We spoke with our senior microbiologist who has assured us that, at this stage, it is highly unlikely that you will suffer from any adverse effects. However we will continue to keep a close eye on you.

PAUSE

'I have also filled out an incident form, which will ensure that the matter will be investigated and steps taken to ensure that it is not repeated.'

ELICIT THE PATIENT'S ONGOING CONCERNS

Mr S: 'But . . . I'm ALLERGIC to penicillin!'

Doctor: 'As I have said, we have now stopped the drug and thankfully you have not suffered any adverse effects. The nursing staff will keep a close eye on you to make sure that you remain well. I again apologise that this has happened. Is there anything in particular that you are still worrying about?'

Mr S: 'It's obvious isn't it? I'm allergic to penicillin. What if I swell up and can't breathe?'

ELICIT PATIENT'S EXPECTATIONS

Doctor: 'At this stage, that is extremely unlikely. Although a delayed reaction is possible, it is rare, and even rarer for you to have a *severe* reaction this late on. I can see that you are still upset about this. Is there anything else that I can do or help you with?'

Mr S: 'I just want to how this happened! I told the nurse at the start I was allergic to penicillin and I want an explanation.'

EMPATHIC RESPONSE

Doctor: 'I appreciate your concerns. Unfortunately when I saw you yesterday I was rushed off my feet and did not document your allergy and as a result you were given the penicillin injection. Although this is not an excuse for what has happened, I have completed an incident form which will mean that this case will be investigated to try to prevent such a mistake from happening again.

PAUSE

'Just to clarify the situation now. We have started you on a different drug for your illness. Once again I and the team are sorry that the mistake has happened.'

FORMAL COMPLAINT	Mr S:	*'I'm still not happy. What if I want to complain? Who do I talk to?'*
	Doctor:	'The hospital has a formal complaints procedure. I am happy to find out some more information for you that will guide you through the process if you so wish.'
	Mr S:	*'I'll think about it.'*
	Doctor:	'Is there anything else I can help you with?'
	Mr S:	*'No. I suppose mistakes can happen and you were very busy yesterday. It seems that you guys are trying to stop it from happening again.'*
SUMMARISE, CLOSE AND AGREE PLAN OF ACTION	Doctor:	'Thanks for appreciating that fact. Would it be alright if I just go over a few things we discussed today?'
	Mr S:	*'Yes, of course.'*
	Doctor:	'When you came in yesterday with pneumonia we started you on antibiotic treatment. Unfortunately, despite the fact that you are allergic to penicillin, you were given two injections of a penicillin-containing drug. Fortunately, you have not reacted badly to these and we have now changed you to a non-penicillin antibiotic.
	PAUSE	
		'I have completed a clinical incident form to ensure that this matter is investigated fully and steps are taken to prevent it from happening again in the future. We have also asked the nurse to keep an eye on you for the next couple of days to make sure there are no delayed reactions. Are you happy with this course of action?'
	Mr S:	*'Yes, Doctor, thank you.'*
	Doctor:	'Thank you for your time, Mr Seeward.'
	CONSULTATION END	

CHAPTER 10

Dealing with complaints

In a consumer-driven society and an NHS in which the emphasis is increasingly on service provision, patients are expecting higher standards of care from doctors and are making complaints more frequently than ever before. Patients who feel they have not received an adequate quality of care have their right to lodge a complaint enshrined in the *Patient's Charter for England*, dating back to 1991.

In the course of your career as a medical professional it is highly likely that you will encounter at least one complaint against you from a patient. Although this may be an extremely distressing event, the manner in which you attempt to resolve the grievance may have a direct bearing on the consequences.

It is a commonly held misconception that the majority of complaints made by patients against the medical establishment are because of failings involving poor care, neglect, clinical negligence or mistakes in diagnosis and treatment. In fact, research indicates that most complaints arise from miscommunication and misunderstandings that occur between the doctor and the patient.

When complaints are made it is easy to allow emotions to gain the better of you. More often than not, this will exacerbate the situation and antagonise the patient further. Hence, good communication with the patient will go some way towards defusing the situation and averting any further action.

The consultation: dealing with complaints

Every complaint, be it written or verbal, should always be acknowledged and taken seriously. Even though you may feel that a patient is being overzealous and unreasonable in their complaint, they are often simply venting their frustration about their care. In complaining, they may feel that in some way things may improve both for themselves and for others in the future.

It is important that you do not allow your emotions to cloud your response but rather adopt a measured and calm approach. Take ample time to prepare yourself with all the facts of the case before entering into consultation with the patient.

Preparation

Before you set out and meet the patient or a relative you should attempt to establish the necessary facts pertaining to the complaint. This may involve you going through the patient's record and summarising the salient points. You may also wish to discuss the complaint with other medical staff who were directly involved in the patient's care. This may shed light and add clarity to the patient's complaint.

When meeting with the patient you should consider the surroundings and organise a suitable time so that you will not be constantly interrupted. On the ward you may consider conducting the meeting in the 'relatives' room'. If possible hand over your bleep to a colleague so that you can free yourself from being disturbed.

Introducing yourself and establishing rapport

How you introduce yourself will help establish good rapport with the patient, which will help create an atmosphere of trust and reduce the risk of the consultation descending into disarray.

In the case of relatives, it is important to establish who you are talking to and their relationship with the patient. Be careful about inadvertently breaching confidentiality when in discussions with relatives. It may be a good idea to gain consent from the patient (if possible) prior to any discussions with their family members.

Acknowledge the patient's complaint

When you are meeting the patient to discuss the complaint you should first acknowledge that the complaint has been received. In so doing, you are demonstrating to the patient that you are taking their views seriously and that you value their opinion. By meeting with them you will automatically assign a sense of formality and show your willingness to correct any mistakes.

Establishing the complaint

It is important to establish the nature of the complaint. Do not assume, for example, that just because a mistake has been made that the complaint is about this. It may be that the patient or relatives are simply unhappy at the way in which things were communicated to them or the way in which the mistake was handled. You may wish to ask the patient:

> 'I understand that you have made a complaint about your treatment on the ward. I would like find about more about this.'

> 'Could you please tell me a little more about what your concerns were?'

By giving the patient a chance to vocalise their concerns you will be able to establish the patient's own understanding about the events surrounding the complaint. This will also provide an opportunity for them to vent any particular frustrations they may have – which may be expressed not only by *what* they say, but also *how* they go about saying it. Don't forget to pick up on any non-verbal cues, such as any change in tone of voice, use of language and general demeanour, as these may provide additional clues as to how the patient is feeling.

In the cases of relatives, it is important to establish their understanding of events. Relatives often come and go on the ward and meet with different staff, so they may gain only snippets of information relating to the patient's care. It is therefore possible that their understanding of events contains factual errors which, once identified, can be easily corrected. Consider the following:

Doctor:	'Hello Mr Wilkins. I understand that you have a complaint regarding aspects of your father's care in hospital. Is this correct?'
Mr Wilkins:	'Well, yes. I know he's had this chest infection and you were giving him injections to treat the blood clot in his lungs. A nurse told me that after only three days he is no longer getting these. How can a blood clot be gone in three days! I know friends who are on treatment for the rest of their lives!'
Doctor:	'I see. Do you mind if I can clarify something with you regarding his treatment?'
Mr Wilkins:	'No, not at all.'
Doctor:	'Your father was admitted to hospital with a chest infection and was quite unwell and not getting out of bed. In such cases we routinely start patients on a low-dose injection to reduce the risk of developing blood clots. Once the patient becomes mobile then they are no longer in need of this. In the case of your father, because he did not show any evidence of blood clots in the lung and he is now mobilising well he no longer needs the injections to thin his blood. Does this help make things clearer?'
Mr Wilkins:	'I see. So when the nurse told me that the injections were for blood clots she meant that they were to prevent them. I understand now! That's cleared that up . . .'

In most cases, such as with the example above, it will be apparent from the complaint as to what the grievance is. You may, however, come across cases where the reason for the complaint is less obvious. In such situations, you may wish to specifically ask the patient or relative to express what their complaint is. Consider the example below:

Mrs Hicks:	'I'm not happy with the care my mother's been receiving.'
Doctor:	'What has been troubling you regarding your mother's care?'
Mrs Hicks:	'Well, ever since she's been in, on a daily basis, doctors have been doing their ward round and, without fail, they have been telling my mother everything that is going on and keeping her fully up to date. I'm not happy.'
Doctor:	'I'm sorry, Mrs Hicks, are you unhappy about the treatment your mother's received?'
Mrs Hicks:	'No, no. I know you've TREATED her right. I'm happy about her overall care, but I'm not happy that she's being told everything.'
Doctor:	'So, you're unhappy that she's been kept informed of her treatment?'
Mrs Hicks:	'Yes.'
Doctor:	'What is your concern regarding this?'
Mrs Hicks:	'I don't want her to be told everything. She gets anxious and worried. I don't want her to know she's ill. I want her to think that she's just in hospital for an MOT and a few tests and that she'll be going home afterwards. She's never been ill before and for you to be telling her all this stuff will only worry her.'

Apology and explanation

Apologise for any hurt caused. Do this even if you feel the complaint was not warranted. This will demonstrate empathy and show that you are sympathetic with the complainant. If the cause for the complaint is a mistake that has been made, apologise for it. Give an account of the events that took place as documented in the medical notes, and explain how things went wrong and what was done to rectify it.

The explanation you give should not aim to be simply a justification of the actions you carried out; rather, it should be an honest attempt to state the chronological order of events as they took place. If a mistake did happen, then inform the patient as to how and why it occurred. You may wish to mention some mitigating circumstances surrounding the mishap, if relevant. Perhaps your team was occupied by an emergency or an acutely unwell patient. There may have been staff absences that hindered communication and despite your aim to provide quality care, lapses had taken place.

You should end your explanation by describing the measures you have taken to rectify things and minimise the damage or hurt caused to the patient. This may lead you on to the patient's or relatives' own expectations about what they hope to occur next.

Doctor:	'I am sorry but I must apologise that your mother was sent home without any medications. It appears that there was a breakdown in communication between the team members. We have just received a new batch of doctors who are still finding their way through the system and it appears, unfortunately, that your mother's drug chart was not taken to the pharmacy. *PAUSE* 'I can assure you that this is not our normal practice. We have taken steps to ensure that it does not happen again.'

Expectations: what does the complainant hope to achieve?

What the patient expects will usually be apparent once you have elicited the nature of the complaint and the concerns surrounding it. For example, a patient who wishes to complain about not having a jug of water at his bedside will probably, following the complaint, want this wish to be fulfilled for the remainder of his stay. However, it is important to bear a few things in mind. Firstly, the patient, in addition to the 'obvious' expectation of having the situation rectified, may wish for something additional that will compensate him for the hurt caused. Consider the following example:

Doctor:	'I am sorry that you have had to endure being next to a disruptive patient. I would like you to know that we have made arrangements for this patient to be moved elsewhere so that you will no longer be troubled. Are you happy with this?'
Patient:	'Well . . . I suppose so . . .'
Doctor:	'Was there something you wanted to add? Please feel free to tell me.'
Patient:	'I don't think it's fair that, because of this lousy patient I've had to put up with, I would have to stay in this bed. I think I deserve a bit more privacy to make up for what I've been put through. I want to be transferred into a side room!'

The above example illustrates how simply taking a problem away may not meet the expectation of certain patients. In these situations, the nature of the consultation will change and become one of negotiation.

Doctor:	'You mentioned, Mr Harris, that you would like to be placed in a separate side room. I appreciate that you have had to endure a difficult period with a noisy and disruptive patient next to you. However, I would like to point out that providing a separate side room may not be possible at the present time.'
Patient:	'Why not? Surely, after everything I've been through, it's the least I deserve.'
Doctor:	'Ideally, every patient would be placed in a separate room of their own. Unfortunately, we don't have enough rooms to go around for everyone, and we are therefore forced to be quite selective as to whom we place in these rooms.'
Patient:	'I've seen that there are at least two rooms for every ward!'
Doctor:	'Most of the time these rooms are used only for patients who have a specific medical reason to go into a side room, perhaps because they have an infection that can be easily spread, and they need to be kept in isolation. Or for a very unwell patient who may be close to death and requires privacy. Unfortunately, we do not have any spare side rooms available – I have checked with the ward manager. *PAUSE* 'We have, however, moved the patient concerned to another location so that you will no longer be disturbed by him. We will continue to try to provide you with the best possible care and cater to your needs. I hope that you understand this.'
Patient:	'Oh, right. I didn't know that's what they were used for. Well, at least he has been moved and I can rest better now!'

The example shows that although the initial expectation of the patient appeared difficult to achieve, with a reasoned explanation, the patient's opinion has been swayed. Most patients are in fact quite understanding and appreciative of the difficulties and dilemmas health professionals face. With an honest and frank discussion, most patients are amenable to reason.

However, in a minority of cases, despite your best efforts, the patient may still decide to take matters further and instigate a formal complaint. In such situations you are obliged to inform them of your local complaints policy and procedures. If you are unaware of these you may wish to seek senior assistance for guidance.

Doctor:	'So, as I have mentioned, we are sorry that this has happened to your father and apologise unreservedly.

	However, the mix up at the laboratory has been rectified and the right treatment has been started. Your father is doing quite well now and we expect him to make a full recovery in the next two days. We have reported this as a clinical incident and it will be investigated fully with action taken to prevent this sort of thing occurring again.'
Relative:	'But my father could have died!'
Doctor:	'I am sorry that this happened. We are taking steps to prevent it from reoccurring. Is there anything else that you would like to see happen?'
Relative:	'I don't know. I'm not happy and I want to take things further.'
Doctor:	'What do you mean, Mr Phillips?'
Relative:	'I don't know. You're the doctor, perhaps I will make a formal complaint.'
Doctor:	'Well, Mr Phillips, it seems that you are still dissatisfied.'
Relative:	'Yes, I am. I want to make an official complaint. How do I go about doing that?'
Doctor:	'Well, I can speak to my senior colleagues and enquire as to how the procedure is started and I will get back to you as soon as I have more information. Is that OK?'
Relative:	'Yes, please. I would like you to do that as soon as possible.'

Summarising back and agreeing on a plan

Having explained the circumstances of the mistake as well as apologising for it you should now agree upon the next course of action. You may have been successful in your attempt to convey to the patient that their complaint has been taken seriously and that necessary steps have been implemented to prevent it from occurring again. In such situations you may wish to summarise back the main points that have been discussed, checking that the patient is still in agreement with you.

Conversely, if despite your efforts the patient still wishes to lodge a formal complaint, you should remain empathic to their position and maintain rapport throughout. Direct them towards the correct departments and offer them assistance in their request.

Closing up and documentation

It is always good practice to ask the patient if they have any other concerns or issues they wish to raise before ending the consultation. If you have agreed a plan of action it may be an appropriate time to conclude the meeting. Thank the patient and offer a follow-up appointment if you feel it is necessary.

Once the patient has left, it is essential that you document what has been discussed, what has been agreed and what course of action has been decided. Whilst it may appear to be a laborious and unrewarding task, these notes may represent the only proof that such discussions have taken place. The patient's notes are a legal document which, if they were to consider taking matters further, would be called as evidence in a court of law.

CLINICAL SCENARIO

Lack of confidentiality

Most complaints arise due to poor communication, a perceived lack of respect, or failing to uphold standards of confidentiality. Such complaints, although appearing to be less important, should not be dismissed and efforts should be made to deal with them at the earliest opportunity. By using effective communication skills you may be able to restore trust and confidence in the patient and avert a potential formal complaint.

DOCTOR'S BRIEF

You are a Foundation Year doctor in Vascular Surgery. This morning, during the ward round, your Consultant was discussing the case of Mr Willis, a 54-year-old man with diabetes. Mr Willis has severe arterial insufficiency of his left lower limb and your Consultant feels that he may need a below-knee amputation in the future. The nurse has informed you that Mr Willis was upset that he could overhear the Consultant's discussion about the amputation from the doctor's room. He is also upset that other patients on the ward have begun to offer him condolences about his impending loss. Your Consultant has gone away on annual leave and is unavailable until late next week. You are the only member of your team available at the moment and the nurse in charge has advised you to have a word with Mr Willis before he is discharged tomorrow.

ACTOR'S BRIEF *(if you are the doctor, please do not read)*

You are Robert Willis, a 54-year-old man with diabetes and longstanding trouble with your legs. You have already faced up to the possibility of having one of your legs amputated. However, you are quite a private person and do not wish others to know about this. You are quite upset that the Consultant has spoken loudly about your problem and that other patients have heard about your possible amputation. You have known your Consultant for some years now, and trust his judgement and believe him to be a good man. More than anything, you are disappointed at him and wish to express your feelings. You have no intention of making a formal complaint, although you have a short temper and cannot stand doctors who don't listen to what you are saying.

SCENARIO WALK-THROUGH

INTRODUCE YOURSELF TO THE PATIENT AND ESTABLISH RAPPORT	*Doctor:*	'Hello, Mr Willis, I'm Dr Jeffers. How are you today?'
	Mr W:	*'Not bad, I suppose.'*
ESTABLISH THE COMPLAINT	*Doctor:*	'The nurse in charge informed me that there was something bothering you. Is that correct?'
	Mr W:	*'Yes, but it was relating to Mr Crawley, the Consultant. I wanted to speak to him personally.'*
	Doctor:	'I'm afraid Mr Crawley is away until next week. Is there anything that I could help you with?'
	Mr W:	*'Well, you obviously know that I'm probably going to have my left leg chopped off. Earlier this morning Mr Crawley was blabbering about it so loudly that I reckon half the hospital heard!'*
	Doctor:	'I see . . .'
	Mr W:	*'Well, I don't want any Tom, Dick or Harry knowing about it! I don't care if you tell the whole world about my diabetes, or about my blood pressure, but not this!'*
CLARIFY THE REASON FOR THE COMPLAINT	*Doctor:*	'So you're upset that others may have heard what the Consultant was saying about your condition?'
	Mr W:	*'Yes. Of course!'*
APOLOGY AND EXPLANATION	*Doctor:*	'First of all, I am sorry that this happened. On behalf of my team, I would like to apologise unreservedly. It is clear that the Consultant's voice was within earshot of other patients. I fully agree that it is not acceptable for anyone to be able to overhear a private discussion regarding a patient.'
	Mr W:	*'So why did it happen?'*
	Doctor:	'I would like to assure you, that there is no doubt that this was an unintentional mistake. We did try to minimise the chance of other people overhearing by using the staff room. However, the door was left open and unfortunately other patients may have overheard the conversation as well.'
	Mr W:	*'So, whose fault is it then? The Consultant, or one of you lot who didn't tell him to quieten down?'*
DO NOT ATTACH OR ACCEPT BLAME	*Doctor:*	'Well, I do not think it is constructive to single out people for blame. However, it is the job of our team

to care for our patients in the best way possible. Obviously a mistake has happened and we will work to make sure that this does not happen again. Once again, I apologise for this occurrence.'

Mr W: *'I see, well obviously you've apologised. But I'm still not very happy.'*

Doctor: 'I appreciate that you are upset about this and that's completely understandable. I plan to let the Consultant know about this when he returns from leave. I will also be organising a meeting with our staff members to ensure our conversations are kept confidential at all times.

PAUSE

EXPLAIN PLAN

'There may be an issue with the set-up of the ward which means that a patient's privacy can be compromised. So, after talking with the Consultant, I will complete an incident form. This means that this episode will be recorded and steps taken to ensure that the same mistake is not repeated. Are you OK with this?'

Mr W: *'Well, all that sounds fine. But I've known Mr Crawley like a friend all these years, and I'm still not 100% happy.'*

ELICIT FURTHER EXPECTATIONS

Doctor: 'Was there something else that you wanted to see happen?'

Mr W: *'I want to speak to the Consultant now. I know he has a mobile number, I would like you to call him now so that I can speak to him.'*

NEGOTIATE

Doctor: 'I appreciate your wish to speak to Mr Crawley now. Unfortunately, it is not possible to arrange such a discussion at the present time. However, I can organise for him to contact you, or for you to make an appointment to see him through his secretary if you would like to see him in person.'

Mr W: *'So when's he coming back?'*

Doctor: 'He will be back at work next Thursday.'

Mr W: *'OK, fair enough. I'd like the number of his secretary and I also want you to personally remind him, in case this all gets lost in red tape.'*

AGREE ON A PLAN	*Doctor:*	'I assure you that when he returns, I will inform him about your concerns and about our discussion so that he is fully aware.'
	Mr W:	*'That sounds like a good idea.'*
ELICIT FURTHER CONCERNS	*Doctor:*	'Was there anything else that you wanted to discuss with me, Mr Willis?'
	Mr W:	*'No, that was the only thing. I just wanted you to be aware of this and let you know how disappointed I was, as I usually get the best quality of care and appreciate it. But I realise that these things happen, and the important thing is that you learn from them.'*
	Doctor:	'If it is OK then, can I just recap on what we have discussed so far to make sure that we are both happy?'
	Mr W:	*'Yes, no problem.'*
SUMMARISE AND CLOSE	*Doctor:*	'This morning, an unfortunate incident happened when patients on the ward were able to overhear a private conversation about your care. Despite the fact that we used the staff room and believed this to be a reasonable precaution, the sound still carried through. We both agree that this was an unfortunate lapse in your care and we are now taking steps to make sure it will not be repeated.
	PAUSE	
		'I will let the Consultant know about this when he returns, and in the meantime you will try to contact his secretary to organise a time to speak to him. Is this OK?'
	Mr W:	*'Yes, it is. Thanks.'*
	Doctor:	'Thank you for your time and understanding, Mr Willis.'
	Mr W:	*'Thank you, Doctor, for taking my concerns on board. I hope that this will not happen again.'*
	CONSULTATION END	

CHAPTER 11

English as a foreign language

Effective communication is the bedrock of the doctor–patient relationship. It is perhaps the most important conduit by which the doctor is able to gain information from the patient about their problems. In most cases, the doctor is able to directly glean the information they require from the patient themselves. However, this is only possible if the two parties converse in the same language.

Increasingly, doctors are finding themselves consulting with patients who are unable to speak English. This situation may raise a number of barriers hindering the consultation. For example, if the patient is unable to adequately express how they feel, they are likely to leave the consultation unfulfilled. However, for the doctor, it may be more hazardous, as a patient may be wrongly diagnosed and incorrectly treated because of miscommunication. It is therefore of utmost importance for the clinician to try to overcome any obstacles that the language barrier may present.

There are several tools a doctor can use to improve communication with patients for whom English is not their first language. The most commonly used of these are interpreter services. However, due to financial and time constraints, they are not always readily available. In fact, with there being just under 7000 languages spoken in the world it is physically impossible to have an interpreter at hand for each and every one. Hence, the onus will be on the doctor to make do with generic verbal and non-verbal communication skills to aid the process. This chapter will focus on some of these techniques and explain how to manoeuvre yourself through this increasingly common challenge.

Interpreters

Interpreters are people who translate orally from one language to another. They play a useful role in facilitating conversation between a clinician and a patient who is unable to speak English. When using an interpreter, the dynamics of the doctor–patient relationship will be distorted from the traditional 'doctor–patient–doctor' to one of, 'doctor–interpreter–patient–interpreter–doctor'.

Interpreters can come in various forms, including professional interpreter services, friends and family members (including children), or telephony services. Each of these has its own benefits and limitations which need to be considered separately.

Professional interpreter services

There are numerous professional interpreting services which employ trained link-workers to interpret for the NHS. By and large, they are committed to a stringent code of ethics which is fully compliant with the principles of the NHS, ensuring trust and confidentiality.

Whilst using an interpreter is an effective way of overcoming language difficulties, it does have some disadvantages. An interpreter may start to analyse what the patient is saying and adapt it to what the doctor wants to hear, thereby changing the meaning of what the patient actually intended. It is also quite easy for the patient to end up becoming the third person in the consultation, with the doctor paying more attention to the interpreter rather than the patient. Consider the following example:

Doctor: 'Can you please ask Mr Zaman what has brought him here today? *(Interpreter poses several questions to Mr Zaman and he answers)*

Interpreter: 'Mr Zaman says he has been suffering from headaches recently.'

Doctor: 'How long has he been having them?' *(Interpreter poses question to Mr Zaman and he answers)*

Interpreter: 'For about one month now. I think it is because of his family problems for the past few months and I believe that is when it started. I heard from my friend . . .'

Doctor: 'What type of family problems?'

Interpreter: 'Well, I heard . . .' *(Mr Zaman twiddles his thumbs whilst Doctor and Interpreter start having a conversation)*

Unfortunately, this type of consultation, where the interpreter becomes the focus of the dialogue, is not uncommon. The doctor may feel more comfortable talking to the interpreter as they both speak the same language. As a result it is more likely that the patient's input about their own problem may be neglected or overlooked.

Relatives

Professional translation services are not always readily available. In such situations the doctor has to rely on alternative solutions such as using the patient's friends or family to translate instead. Such translators may not have had any formal training or assessments of their competency in English. As a result the interpreter's level of understanding and ability to communicate may be limited. Other problems that may arise with their use may include a breach of confidentiality and potential embarrassment when discussing sensitive matters. This makes the use of such translators a matter of necessity rather than standard practice.

Consider the example below whereby a patient visits his GP complaining of testicular pain whilst his friend acts as a stand-in interpreter:

Doctor: 'I have examined you quite thoroughly and I couldn't feel any obvious lumps or bumps down below. In fact, I wasn't able to elicit any of that tenderness you described to me.'
(Patient's friend translates throughout)

Patient: 'OK, Doctor. That's fine.'
(Still looks a little restless and agitated)

Doctor: 'Mr Rodriguez, you still seem to be a little worried. Is there anything else you would like to talk to me about?'

Patient: 'No, thank you.'

Doctor: 'Mr Rodriguez, everything we do talk about strictly remains between us. By telling me exactly what is worrying you, I can try to give you the help you need. You seem to be quite agitated. Why don't you tell me what is bothering you?'

Patient: 'Thank you, Doctor. I am fine. Can I have another appointment in two weeks' time?'

Doctor: 'OK. I'll book a double appointment and make sure we have an NHS interpreter.'
(Patient returns for his follow-up appointment)

Doctor: 'You seemed quite worried last week. Was there anything you wanted to talk about in private?'
(Professional interpreter translates)

Patient: 'Thank you, doctor. The thing is, a few weeks ago I had sex with a prostitute. I'd never usually do such a thing, and I've always been dead against such acts. I don't know why I did it. But now I'm really worried that I may have caught some sort of infection.'
(Professional interpreter continues to translate . . .)

Telephony

If nobody is physically available to help translate, you may consider using a telephone translation service to get through the consultation. These function by the doctor ringing a company and booking a translator for a specific language. The company rings back once a translator is found. The doctor will then feed their questions to the interpreter before passing the handset to the patient for a response.

Telephone translations are a new field that most doctors have yet to have training in. They are likely to throw up new problems in an already difficult consultation. By using a telephone, your focus may be distracted from the patient and from any non-verbal cues they may express. In addition, the interpreter provides a literal translation of what the patient has said and is unable to appreciate or note any non-verbal cues from the other party. Subsequently, there is potential for key points and subtleties to be missed in the conversation.

Absence of interpreter

Frequently, none of the above options are available to the doctor. You may find yourself staring at a patient who understands hardly any English at all. The patient may be unwell, in need of urgent assessment, or simply be unwilling to leave having waited a few hours to see you. Whatever the circumstances, you will need to improvise using a variety of verbal and non-verbal communication skills to gain the most you can from this awkward situation.

Verbal skills

Try your best to avoid any jargon or complex idioms that the patient is unlikely to understand. Instead, keep your sentences short and simple to avoid unnecessary confusion.

Doctor: 'I think the pain in your abdomen is because of a possible obstructed inguinal hernia. You will need to see a colorectal surgeon who may have to perform an open laparotomy in hospital.'

Patient: *(Confused)* 'Me no understand no English. Who is Mr Hernia?'

When talking to the patient, it may be helpful to use ubiquitous words that transcend different languages and are generally well understood; words such as 'chemist', 'antibiotics', or 'paracetamol', may help the patient's understanding. It may also be useful to repeat specific points so that the patient is afforded more opportunities to grasp the gist of the conversation. You should also speak more slowly and articulate your words clearly to aid communication.

You may be tempted to project your voice more loudly in the hope that the non-English speaking individual may understand you better. By doing so, you are more likely to appear as aggressive and intimidating, so much so that insurmountable barriers are created.

Doctor:	*(Bellowing)* 'DO YOU SPEAK ENGLISH?'
Patient:	*(Alarmed)* 'Non. Me no English.'
Doctor:	'WHAT DO YOU WANT FROM ME TODAY . . .?'
Patient:	'Huh *(Shuddering)* . . . no problem, no problem. Me go home?'

Non-verbal skills

When trying to communicate information to a non-English speaking patient, you will probably find that you have to rely more on your non-verbal communication skills. There are universally recognised facial expressions as well as hand gestures that convey the same meaning across all languages and cultures. A patient in pain or concern can easily be identified by their grimace. Locating the source of pain can be done through gesturing. Likewise, a simulated cough, sneeze or a retch can be easily demonstrated and equally understood.

Try to remain attentive as well as encouraging towards the patient, particularly when they struggle to respond to your questions. The more the patient relaxes and feels your empathy, the more likely they will be able to communicate their concerns and worries to you. Simple things such as nodding your head, saying: *'Yes, go on . . .'* as well as having an open posture, can be constructive to the consultation. Avoid being condescending or dismissive in your attitude towards the patient as this is likely to upset them.

Props

You may consider using commonly available props to prompt your way through the consultation. Simple things, such as a pen and paper, a calendar or an analogue clock, can be used to good effect, particularly when explaining drug dosage, frequency and times of use. Diagrams drawn with basic instructions can be taken away by the patient and if necessary, translated later on by a friend or family member.

The consultation: preparation

Before meeting the patient, try to identify whether you will need an interpreter, and if so, for which language. Occasionally, the patient may attend with a friend or family member who is able to speak some English. Whilst they should not be discouraged from attending, the doctor should still insist on the presence of a professional interpreter if available and only use the family member as a fallback should this not be possible.

Pay attention to the layout of the consultation room as it can get quite crowded. Ensure that there are extra chairs so that no one is left standing awkwardly. Try to position yourself in close proximity to the patient away from any obstacles, such as a desk, that may obstruct your line of vision.

When communicating, direct your questions at the patient and observe them for any non-verbal cues. Keep any translators in the background and focus your attention solely on the patient. Consider allowing extra time when conducting such consultations – it might be sensible to put such appointments towards the end of the patient list or to book double appointments.

Introduction and establishing rapport

The initial stage of the consultation can be a daunting prospect for both the doctor and the patient. From the patient's perspective, the uncertainty and unfamiliarity associated with a consultation in a foreign language can be quite frightening. For the doctor, having to conduct a consultation with a patient who cannot speak their language can be very frustrating. By getting the consultation off to a good start, these early apprehensions can be significantly reduced.

Invite the patient into the room which ideally has already been prepared. Greet them with a simple hello or even a handshake if appropriate. State your name and designation whilst pointing to yourself to make it clear who you are. Ask the patient who they are and what language they speak. Try to ascertain whether or not they understand English to a good degree before trying to locate an interpreter.

Purpose of the consultation

Elicit the main problems and concerns that the patient has come to see you about. Use appropriate communication techniques, as described as above, to help understand the purpose of their visit.

When enquiring about symptoms, point to parts of the body, such as the head, neck, chest and abdomen, so that the patient can indicate the anatomical site of concern.

Doctor: 'I am Dr Johnson *(Doctor points to self)*. What is your name?' *(Doctor points to patient)*

Mei Lay Chun: 'Me no speak English well. Interpreter?'

Doctor: 'OK, OK. Which language do you speak?' *(Doctor points to mouth)*

Mei Lay Chun: 'Mandarin.'
(Doctor contacts receptionist and attempts to find Mandarin interpreter)

Doctor: 'Sorry, no interpreter today. How can I help you?'
(Doctor points to self then points to patient)

Mei Lay Chun: 'Pain.' *(Patient points to tummy)*

Ideas, concerns and expectations

Trying to establish the ideas, concerns and expectations of the non-English speaking patient is just as important as for any other patient. However, you may find that achieving this feat will be a lot more taxing. If you have a professional interpreter present this task may be lessened, particularly if they have had previous health training. In such circumstances, you should ask the patient their own ideas about their symptoms and any concerns or worries that they may possess.

In those situations where an interpreter is not present, an attempt should still be made at establishing the patient's thoughts as to their symptoms. There is no easy way of doing this other than asking the patient directly. Their response may be hindered by the degree of English they understand and are able to speak.

Doctor: 'What do you think is the cause of your headaches?'
Patient: 'Sorry?'
Doctor: *(Doctor speaks slowly)* 'Why do you have headache?'
Patient: 'Headache? Pain all the time. My dad *(Points to head)* cancer.'

History

Attempt to take as full a history as possible from the patient with regard to their presenting complaint. Try to ask all the usual associated questions, such as when it started, how long it has been present, how severe and any other concurrent symptoms. You will have to use all your communication skills to their full potential in order to gain a detailed picture of what is going on. It can be easy to forget to use your non-verbal communication skills, such as miming, looking for cues and understanding, and using facial expressions. If necessary, use any props to your advantage, such as a calendar to determine when the symptom started and how long it has gone on for. There are now a number of visual scales depicting symptoms such as pain and its increasing severity that you may find useful. Show these to the patient and allow them to choose a picture to represent how bad their pain is.

Try completing your medical history by going on to ask about the patient's drug, family and social history. Pointing to tablets and asking if they take any medication may prompt the patient to reveal them. You may wish to ask about drug allergies by miming the taking of a tablet and scratching oneself immediately afterwards. Alcohol intake may be determined by mimicking the action of drinking, whilst smoking history can be ascertained by pretending to smoke a cigarette.

Summarise back to the patient at regular intervals to ensure that they understood what has been asked.

Examination and diagnosis

In a real-life situation you would complete your assessment by offering to examine the patient and undertake any relevant investigations or procedures. In the exam setting it is highly unlikely that you would be asked to perform this task in addition to taking a very difficult and challenging history. More likely, you will be expected to explain your working diagnosis and management plan to the patient.

Management

Once the patient has been told of their diagnosis, it is important to discuss with them the possible treatment options. These may include a referral for further investigations, specialist review or providing a prescription for medication. Miscommunication for any of these may be problematic, but particularly so for drug therapy. Any misunderstanding of dosage regime may cause direct harm through overdosing or result in inadequate treatment through underdosing.

Doctor: 'Because of the blood clot in your leg you have to take this tablet called warfarin to thin the blood. On weekdays you need to take 4 mg and weekends 3 mg. To make up the 4 mg tablets you should take a 3 mg tablet and a 1 mg tablet together. Is that clear?'

Patient: 'OK, doctor. I eat four tablets when I have pain. Ya?'

As we can see from the above example, the doctor appears to have rushed through their explanation of the treatment leaving the patient bewildered and confused. They may be at risk of harming themselves as a result. A more helpful approach would be to, firstly, use simple words and terms that the patient may understand. Secondly, present your explanation in a sequential and logical fashion. Finally, check the patient's understanding at key points during your explanation. A simple thumbs-up or a casual nod of the head is a internationally understood way of checking if everything is OK and the patient is happy with what you have told them.

Using props

It is not always easy to articulate and convey complex concepts to a patient who *does* speak English, let alone to someone for whom English is not their first language. It may be an idea to facilitate your communication by using common props at your disposal.

Simple props, such as a pen and paper, can be used to illustrate timings when medications should be taken. The drawing of organs and bodily systems can be used to show disease or dysfunction. Also, simple written instructions can be taken away by the patient to act as a reference and reinforce what has been said.

Other items, such as a wall clock or watch, can often help to describe the exact time medication should be taken, whilst a calendar can be used to show treatment length or dates for future appointments.

Doctor:	'For the blood clot in your leg you need to take tablets to make it better. Do you understand?'
Patient:	'Yes. Big leg need tablet.'
Doctor:	'This tablet helps makes the blood thin and move better in the leg.'
Patient:	'OK.'
Doctor:	'You need to take two tablets together from Monday to Friday . . . *(Doctor points out days on calendar)* 'Take the brown coloured one (1 mg tablet) and the blue coloured one (3 mg tablet) together. 'At weekends – Saturday take one blue tablet and Sunday take one blue tablet. Is that OK?'
Patient:	'Can I have paper?'
Doctor:	'OK. Let me write it out clearly so you can take it with you.'

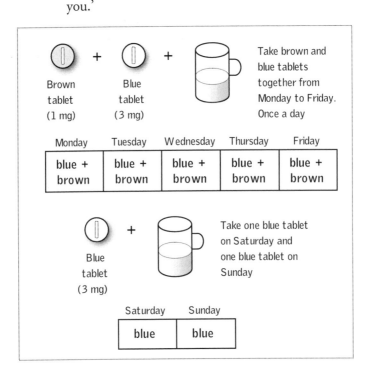

Follow-up

Follow-up for such consultations is extremely important, particularly if you did not have access to an interpreter. By booking a follow-up appointment you can give yourself ample time to arrange a professional translator and organise a double appointment for the patient. It will also allow you an opportunity to check the patient's understanding of what was said previously and check symptom resolution.

You should make every effort to book the appointment before the patient leaves your room to avoid any confusion regarding timing or dates. Give them an appointment card, with your name clearly stated, to take away with them. Use a calendar if necessary to illustrate the date of the follow-up appointment.

Closing up

After a difficult consultation you may still feel that the patient has not understood you despite your efforts. It may be an idea to make use of additional resources such as translated patient information leaflets which can be printed off and given to the patient. If taken from a trusted site, these will often mirror much of what you have already told the patient and reinforce key concepts. Often the English version is also available for you to read to check that you are happy with its content.

Close the consultation by thanking the patient and reminding them to attend their follow-up. This can be communicated non-verbally by either offering your hand for a handshake or walking them to the door.

CLINICAL SCENARIO

Patient with a sore throat

When speaking to a patient who does not communicate well in English it is important that you try to simplify your speech to help communication. Avoid falling into the trap of giving overly complicated and long-winded advice which can lead to confusion and misunderstanding in the patient. Look out for any props or items that can be used to facilitate the consultation.

DOCTOR'S BRIEF

You are one of the GP Registrars. You have been asked to see a patient who is new to the locality, and has just registered with the practice. However, the receptionist has informed you that the patient speaks little English, and it is difficult to arrange for an interpreter at such short notice. Obtain a history from the patient and advise accordingly.

ACTOR'S BRIEF *(if you are the doctor, please do not read)*

You are Li Chua. You have just moved to the locality, and have registered with your nearest GP practice. Your native tongue is Vietnamese and you speak very little English. In fact, you have been in this country for only the last three months. You have recently developed a sore throat with mild changes to your voice. You are quite concerned, as you have had a nasty infection in the past which required antibiotics. You have come here expecting to receive a script for antibiotics again.

SCENARIO WALK-THROUGH

INTRODUCE YOURSELF TO THE PATIENT AND ESTABLISH RAPPORT	*Doctor:* 'Hello. My name is Dr Bateman. How can I help you today?'
	Ms Chua: *'My name Li Chua. Me speak no English.'*
ESTABLISH PATIENT DOES NOT SPEAK ENGLISH	*Doctor:* 'What language do you speak?'
	Ms Chua: *'Vietnamese. Reception say no interpret.'*
DON'T BE CONDESCENDING OR DISMISSIVE TOWARDS THE PATIENT	*Doctor:* 'Fine. Take a seat. *(Doctor gestures to sit down)* What seems to be the problem?'
	Ms Chua: *'Pain here.' (Patient rubs throat)*
ELICIT PROBLEMS USING GESTURING AS APPROPRIATE	*Doctor:* 'When did it start?'
	Ms Chua: *'Huh?'*
USE PROPS TO GAIN A MORE DETAILED HISTORY	*Doctor:* 'Start? One day back? Two day back?'
	(Doctor points to calendar)
	Ms Chua: *'Two day back.'*
USE MIMING	*Doctor:* 'Pain on moving neck?' *(Doctor flexes and extends his neck)*
	Ms Chua: *'No.' (Patient mimics Doctor's movements)*
	Doctor: 'Runny nose?' *(Doctor blows his nose)*
	Ms Chua: *'Yes ... yes ...'*
	Doctor: 'Temperature?' *(Doctor flaps his hand like a fan besides his face)*
	Ms Chua: *'Yes last night very hot.'*
	Doctor: 'Can I look?' *(Doctor points own finger to his eye then to patient's throat)*
	Ms Chua: *'OK.'*
	(Doctor begins to examine the patient)
EXPLAIN DIAGNOSIS IN CLEAR SIMPLE TERMS	*Doctor:* 'I have checked your throat *(Doctor points to throat)*, your ears *(Doctor points to ears)* and your chest *(Doctor points to chest)*. You have a small viral infection, not big. For a small infection, paracetamol is a good tablet. You can buy it from a chemist.'
	Ms Chua: *'No antibiotic?'*

ELICIT PATIENT'S EXPECTATIONS AND ADDRESS PATIENT'S CONCERNS	

Doctor: 'Antibiotics only good for big infections like bacteria. Antibiotics no good in small viral infections. Antibiotic will not help.'

Ms Chua: *'Old doctor give me antibiotic!'*

GIVE PATIENT INSTRUCTIONS ON WHAT TO DO AND WHEN TO COME BACK IF NOT IMPROVED	

Doctor: 'This time infection is small and no need for antibiotic. Take paracetamol for two days and if no good come back.'

Ms Chua: *'Take paracetamol then come back?'*

Doctor: 'If good after two days no need to come back. Try to rest *(Doctor gestures sleeping position)* and drink lots of water *(gestures drinking motion)*. If still no good come back, OK?'

Ms Chua: *'OK. How many paracetamol?'*

EXPLAIN MEDICATION DOSAGE USING PROPS IF NECESSARY	

Doctor: 'Take two tablets four times a day. Take two tablets at breakfast, two at lunch, two at dinner and two before sleeping.' *(Doctor explains this by drawing pictures)*

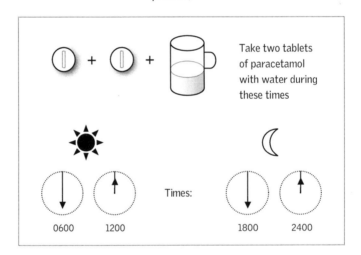

Ms Chua: *'So two 6 o'clock, two 12 o'clock, two evening, two night time.'*

Doctor: 'Yes, that's it.'

Ms Chua: *'Where I get paracetamol?'*

Doctor: 'Go to the chemist.'

Ms Chua: *'OK, thank you.'*

CHECK PATIENT'S UNDERSTANDING	
SUMMARISE BACK	

Doctor: 'Are you happy with what I say to you?'

Ms Chua: 'Yes.'

Doctor: 'You tell me what I said to you?'

Ms Chua: *'Yes, my neck problem is little infection. Antibiotic no work. I take paracetamol for two days. I rest and drink more water. If not better I come to see you after two days?'*

Doctor: 'Yes, very good. OK, Ms Chua, goodbye.' *(Doctor offers handshake and follows patient to door)*

Ms Chua: *'Goodbye now.'*

CONSULTATION END

CHAPTER 12

Prejudices and discrimination

As doctors, you will encounter a wide range of people from different backgrounds and cultures during your professional careers. These people may live quite varied and colourful lifestyles, and hold beliefs or practices that may not necessarily be in harmony with your own. There may even be times when the patient's beliefs may directly oppose particular beliefs that you hold dear. This predicament should not be allowed to interfere with how you go about treating and managing your patient. You should recall the moment when you qualified as a doctor and promised to treat all people equally according to the Hippocratic Oath, '*I will treat without exception all who seek my ministrations, so long as the treatment of others is not compromised thereby*'.

Doctors, like everyone else, inevitably have their own opinions and perceptions about different groups and individuals. These may be formed as a result of past experience, due to religious beliefs or even stem from hearsay or conjecture. More often than not, people's ideas and opinions are derived from depictions in the media, which can be misrepresent and be ill-informed, creating stereotypes. When such stereotypes are acted upon or cause a change in behaviour towards an individual, this is known as discrimination and the person acting this way is prejudiced.

Prejudice can be defined as holding a preconceived idea, judgement or belief towards an individual or group of people because of their ethnicity, gender, age, class, religion or other specific characteristics. In the context of the medical profession, holding a prejudice may mean a doctor assuming something about a patient that is incorrect and allowing this assumption to cloud or affect their judgement towards them. In essence, a patient is discriminated against and treated differently simply because of a prejudice held against them.

Discrimination

Although prejudice may simply be a belief or opinion that you hold, when it unfairly affects your judgement towards an individual it is known as discrimination. Discrimination may manifest simply as a change in attitude towards the patient, or be more insidious, such as reducing access to services or withholding treatment altogether.

There are numerous studies that have shown disparity between the quality of healthcare of ethnic minorities compared with the indigenous (or dominant) population. Other studies highlight a tendency to more actively treat and engage with the higher social economic classes as opposed to the working class and the unemployed.

When most people think of discrimination in the health sector they think of overt forms, such as withholding expensive treatment from the elderly due to an assumption that it is not 'cost effective'. However, subtle forms of prejudice are more common, such as believing unemployed patients are feigning illness to get statutory sick pay.

Although no one is immune from holding prejudices, you should make every attempt to reflect on your own behaviour and try to prevent your prejudices from interfering with your medical judgement and performance.

The consultation

Prejudices may arise even before the patient sets foot into the consulting room. A doctor may have access to the patient's notes detailing their name, age, gender, ethnicity and sexual orientation. This information has the potential to trigger prejudices in the mind of the doctor before even meeting the patient. Although these details are important, you should be careful not to form any assumptions regarding the patient at this stage.

Prejudices may also manifest when the patient enters the room. Their skin colour, appearance, speech and mannerisms may arouse a deep-seated prejudice and cause you to discriminate against them.

When a doctor holds a prejudice against a patient, for whatever reason, it may become apparent to the patient during the consultation. It may be quite obvious – in the form of your facial expression, such as being startled, shocked or frowning – or more subtle, through the tone of your voice or the haste with which you end the consultation. You may even become dismissive, obstructive and adopt a closed posture towards the patient. All of these cues can be picked up by the patient and may cause offence.

Consider the following example of an Asian woman who has come to see the Psychiatrist regarding treatment for her son's newly diagnosed schizophrenia.

Doctor:	'So, you understand that your son has been diagnosed with paranoid schizophrenia?'
Mother:	'Yes.'
Doctor:	'What do you know about the illness?'

Mother:	'Well, actually my priest believes my son has been taken over by evil spirits.'
Doctor:	*(Doctor tuts)* 'I see . . . well, isn't it better to take your son to the priest then instead of wasting my time?!'
Mother:	'But . . . aren't you going to do anything to help?'
Doctor:	*(Annoyed)* 'Well, what can I do if your son has been possessed as you say? Who do you think I am? I'm a medical healer, not a spiritual healer!'

Different types of prejudices

Prejudices against people are commonly held on grounds such as race and ethnicity, gender, age, sexual orientation, and religious beliefs. Below we will consider a few examples of these.

Race and ethnicity

Probably the most commonly held prejudice in society is one against race, ethnicity and skin colour. Some people may assume that individuals of a certain race or ethnicity are less intelligent, poorly spoken and unskilled. One may go further and associate certain behaviours, such as drug taking, gun crime and criminal activity, with specific ethnic groups. Consider the following example of Mr Jermaine Walsh, a 19-year-old African–Caribbean man who attends his local casualty department after sustaining a large gash to his forearm. The doctor notices he is wearing a baseball cap and several gold rings on each hand.

Doctor:	'Hello, I'm Dr Jones. Are you Mr Walsh?'
Mr W:	'Yes.'
Doctor:	'I understand you've injured your arm?'
Mr W:	'Yeah, there's a big cut there.'
Doctor:	'When did it happen?'
Mr W:	'This evening.'
Doctor:	'Do you know what caused it?'
Mr W:	'Well, actually . . .'
Doctor:	'It looks like a knife wound. Were you attacked with a knife?'
Mr W:	'No. I was just in the garage . . .'
Doctor:	'This area, unfortunately, has noticed a lot of gang crime recently and I have seen my fair share of stabbings.'
Mr W:	'I am not part of any gangs. You got me all wrong . . .'
Doctor:	'Don't worry everything you tell me today is held in the strictest of confidence.'

Mr W:	'No, Doc. It's not what you think.'
Doctor:	'You were lucky you were not shot. I've seen a lot young lives wasted because of this!'
Mr W:	'That's it! I'm going somewhere else!'

Other ethnic groups are often tainted with different brushes. Asian families may be assumed to be involved in consanguineous marriages from overseas, whilst Roma people may be unfairly associated with truancy, unemployment and lacking fixed abode. Consider the following case of an Irish man who attends his GP with a history of epigastric pain.

Doctor:	'So, you've been having this pain just under your chest bone for several months?'
Patient:	'Yes, Doctor.'
Doctor:	'And what makes it worse?'
Patient:	'It seems to get worse after a heavy meal or when I am hungry.'
Doctor:	'And after a drink?'
Patient:	'I don't drink, Doctor.'
Doctor:	'You're Irish, correct?'
Patient:	'Yes, Doctor.'
Doctor:	'And you don't drink? I am sure you have a tipple now and then.' *(Laughing)*
Patient:	'No, Doctor. I don't touch the stuff!'
Doctor:	'Come on. Not even on St Patrick's Day?'
Patient:	'Pardon me?'

In the example above the doctor's mistake was not his initial suspicion that alcohol could play a major factor in this patient's symptoms. Rather, it was his insistence on believing that the patient drank alcohol because of his ethnicity.

Gender

Despite it being almost 100 years since the Suffragettes managed to gain the right for women to vote, gender discrimination still plays a prominent part in today's society. Women are still perceived to be less intelligent than their male counterparts, indecisive and governed by their emotions. It is still a commonly held belief that women's place is in the home performing household chores and looking after the children.

Consider this example of a 36-year-old woman who attends her GP complaining of pain in her upper limbs.

Doctor:	'Hello Miss Tate. What can I do for you today?'

Patient:	'I've been having these pains in my arms, particularly in the hands and fingers.'
Doctor:	'I see. How long has this been going on for?'
Patient:	'For about three to four months. It started off happening at any time but now it occurs mainly in the evening.'
Doctor:	'Hmm. Is it made worse when you're carrying the kids or changing them?'
Patient:	'I'm sorry? What kids?'
Doctor:	'I mean your family . . . your children.'
Patient:	'What children? I don't have any children. I work full time in IT.'
Doctor:	'Oh . . . You're cutting it a bit fine, aren't you?'
Patient:	'I don't understand what you saying? How is that related to my pains?'
Doctor:	'The computer says you are 36 years old. Don't you know that as you get older your fertility drops and makes it more difficult for you to conceive?'

In this example, the doctor's assumption that a woman aged 36 should have children has completely digressed from the patient's presenting complaint. The patient is taken aback by the doctor's line of questioning and is likely to feel offended by his comments. The patient's reasons for not having children are entirely personal and have no role to play in this consultation.

Age

Age is another factor which is commonly discriminated against. Elderly people are almost universally thought of as being confused, dependent and in need of carers. When speaking to them, most people will raise their voice believing that they are also hard of hearing. Unfortunately, they are also thought to be at 'death's door' with any money spent on them being not 'cost effective'. As a result, a number of treatment options may be unfairly withheld.

In the following example, a 76-year-old man attends his local casualty department presenting with a large bruise on his head.

Doctor:	*(BELLOWS)* 'Hello, Mr Jenkins, I'm Dr Williams. Oh dear, what have you done to yourself.'
Patient:	'I'm not entirely sure, Doctor . . .'
Doctor:	*(BELLOWS)* 'Where is your hearing aid? Can you hear me alright?'
Patient:	'No need to shout, I can hear you perfectly well!'
Doctor:	'Not to worry, my dear sir. Oh dear! Oh dear! What a nasty bruise. So, how did you fall at home, sir? Was it down the stairs?'

Patient:	'I didn't have a fall.'
Doctor:	'Of course you haven't, of course. Perhaps you don't remember? People often don't remember these things at your age. Don't worry we'll soon have you patched up and back in front of the fireplace.'
Patient:	'I'm telling you I didn't fall over!'
Doctor:	'It's alright, Mr Jenkins, you're in safe hands now. Do you know where you are?'
Patient:	'Yes, of course I do. I'm in St John's hospital, London. I took the 62 bus down here.'
Doctor:	'And do you know who I am?'
Patient:	'You are Dr Williams. Are you having a laugh?'
Doctor:	'That's very good, Mr Jenkins. I see you are quite a witty old thing. No it's not a joke. It's alright to be a little bit muddled at your age.'
Patient:	'What on earth are you talking about? I'm not confused at all. I'd like to speak to someone in charge. I'm perfectly fine. I was brought here after something hit me whilst I was on the seventeenth hole at the golf club. I'm not sure if it was a ball or the swing of a club . . .'

By the time the truth has come out and the doctor has finally learnt that his patient is not cognitively impaired and is in fact an extremely fit and active 76-year-old, the doctor–patient relationship has been damaged beyond repair.

At the other end of the age spectrum, young people (particularly youths and adolescents) are often stigmatised and portrayed as being unemployed and uneducated. In addition, they may be assumed to be involved in gangs and criminal activities. The media also renders them as being promiscuous and involved in risky social behaviours such as drug taking and binge drinking.

Consider the example of this 16-year-old Caucasian girl complaining of thrush-like symptoms.

Doctor:	'What seems to be the problem?'
Patient:	'I'm getting itching down below, and this cheesy whitish discharge. It's really irritating me. I've had thrush several times before and I think I've got it again.'
Doctor:	'I see. I'm going to have to ask you a few personal questions about it.'
Patient:	'OK.'
Doctor:	'How many sexual partners have you had recently?'

Patient:	'None actually!'
Doctor:	'Are you sure?'
Patient:	'Yes.'
Doctor:	'Are you sure it's just itchiness and the discharge? Is there nothing else?'
Patient:	'Yes. There's nothing else, Doctor.'
Doctor:	'I just want to reassure you that everything you say is confidential. It is fine to tell me how many partners you have slept with.'
Patient:	'I've told you, I'm not in a relationship at the moment. I haven't even had sex yet!'

It is evident that in the example above, the doctor has assumed that there is more to the patient's symptoms than what she is letting on. Even though the patient repeatedly denies this, the doctor persists in pursuing this line of questions. His assumptions have caused him to fail to ask important questions relating to thrush and adopt a very narrow approach in taking the history.

Religion

Religious discrimination usually takes the form of incorrect assumptions about what a person believes. Misconceptions are common, because although most people know something about the practices of the main religions, not all adherents strictly follow these religious precepts. Common misconceptions include believing all Muslims and Hindus have forced or arranged marriages, that Jews do not permit autopsy on their deceased, and that Christians refuse blood transfusions.

Consider the case below whereby a 25-year-old Muslim woman attends her GP with a facial bruise.

Doctor:	'Right, Mrs Khan. Can you tell me how you sustained that bruise to your face?'
Patient:	'Oh, it's nothing. I just slipped on the rug yesterday.'
Doctor:	'Really? It looks like a quite nasty bruise to me. I am not sure that a simple fall can explain it.'
Patient:	'But that's what happened, Doctor.'
Doctor:	'Didn't your parents marry you off recently, abroad?'
Patient:	'Well, I did get married. But in this country and to someone I chose.'
Doctor:	'As you know I am here to help. Whatever you tell me will remain within these four walls.'
Patient:	'Yes, I know that . . .'

Doctor:	'I can only help you if you tell me what REALLY happened.'
Patient:	'I am not sure what you are talking about?'
Doctor:	'I understand it may be a stigma in your community to talk about these things. If you change your mind you are more than welcome to come back and see me. In the meantime if it happens again here is the domestic violence helpline for you to call.'

Whilst domestic violence is an issue that blights society at large, the doctor incorrectly assumed this Muslim woman's bruise was due to it. Again, the doctor has completely ignored the patient's problem and broached an extremely sensitive matter tactlessly. In so doing, he is likely to have incensed the patient and may have deterred her from seeking medical advice from him at a later date.

Sexual orientation

Prejudices have been held against people of different sexual orientations for many centuries. Although such prejudice is most often directed at homosexuals it can, less commonly, be against heterosexuals. Predominant stereotypes include assuming that such people are more promiscuous, engage in risk-taking behaviour and have increased incidence of sexually transmitted infections, including HIV.

Consider the example of a 35-year-old man attending with his partner, to the GP.

Doctor:	'Hello, Mr Williams. Come in and take a seat. Your friend can sit over there . . . 'How can I help you today?'
Patient:	'It's a bit embarrassing. I am experiencing pain after doing a number two.'
Doctor:	'I see. Are you sure you want to discuss this in front of your friend? Maybe it is an idea if your friend waits outside?'
Patient:	'Don't worry it is OK. He is my partner.'
Doctor:	'Sorry?'
Patient:	'He is my boyfriend. We got married recently.'
Doctor:	'Oh . . . OK. Err . . . hmm . . . Perhaps you can try some lactulose. It's a bit busy today so I won't be examining you. If it doesn't get better you can go to the local sexual health clinic.'

Undoubtedly, certain practices or lifestyles may seem shocking to many people. As doctors, however, it is not our role to judge these or to allow our own personal beliefs to affect our judgement when treating such patients.

Lifestyle: smoking and alcohol

Taking a history of alcohol and tobacco use is often an important part of the consultation. Prejudice in these areas often relates to assumptions regarding habits and consumption, particularly in certain social classes. It may be assumed that a social smoker or drinker is equally as blameworthy for their illness as a heavy smoker or binge drinker.

Consider the case of a 20-year-old student who is found to have elevated liver enzymes and is called in by his GP for an appointment to discuss the results.

Doctor: 'A recent blood test has shown that you have had some damage to your liver. I need to ask you some questions about your health. How much alcohol do you drink?'

Patient: 'Maybe one or two pints at the weekend.'

Doctor: 'Right. I see. I've been a student myself and I know how much you guys can drink. Your blood tests show your liver is currently working too hard. It's best just to be honest with me and tell me how much you really drink.'

Patient: 'No, seriously. I only drink one or two pints during the football on Saturdays. Sometimes not even that.'

Doctor: 'What about when you go clubbing? Surely you get plastered each time?'

Patient: 'I don't go clubbing, loud music just gives me a headache.'

Doctor: 'Oh come on. You're a student for God's sake! Now tell me, how often do you go on a binge, or a pub-crawl?'

Patient: 'Never have, never will.'

Doctor: 'Well, until you face up to the fact that you have an alcohol problem we can't help you. Now, do you use alcohol in the morning as an eye opener?'

It may be tempting to be judgemental about patients who suffer from diseases or illnesses that are perceived to be caused by lifestyle choices. One may be less empathic and more accusatory towards the patient implicating their lifestyle as the primary cause of their medical problems.

Consider the example of a 50-year-old patient suffering from COPD and complaining of shortness of breath.

Doctor: 'I've just done your spirometry reading and it shows that

	you suffer from chronic lung disease. The main cause of this is smoking. Do you smoke, sir?'
Patient:	'Yes, I do. I have been smoking 40 a day.'
Doctor:	'For how long?'
Patient:	'Almost 35 years.'
Doctor:	'Good God. Don't you know what you have done to your lungs, smoking like a chimney?'
Patient:	'Well, I've been trying to quit. I have cut down recently.'
Doctor:	'Well, it's all too little, too late. What do you expect me to do now? The chances are that you will need oxygen for the rest of your life. You are probably well on your way to getting lung cancer.'
Patient:	'Oh no . . .'

Tackling prejudices

Most people hold ideas and beliefs that are dear to themselves – on a wide range of issues, such as God, religion, politics, lifestyle and behaviours. As doctors, our primary duty is the health of our patients irrespective of their background or lifestyle choices. This has been clearly stated in the GMC guidance entitled *The Duties of the Doctor*, that proclaims as a doctor you must '*make the care of your patient your first concern*', as well as '*make sure that your personal beliefs do not prejudice your patients' care*'.

Prejudice can adversely affect the consultation in many ways. The doctor may make incorrect assumptions about the patient, examples of which have been outlined above. It also may push the doctor to use inappropriate language and mannerisms towards the patient thus causing stress, offence and ill feeling. More seriously, however, prejudice may lead to discrimination by affecting clinical judgement and restricting treatment options.

Being aware of common prejudices will allow you to empathise with the experiences these individuals encounter on a regular basis. It will also permit you to recognise and accept diversity in the different lifestyles, beliefs and habits that you may encounter. This may also help you overcome any personal prejudices you may harbour.

When consulting with such patients, you should always keep the patient's care as your main focus and concern. Use open questions where possible and explore sensitive topics in a tactful, non-judgemental way. By doing so you will help the patient relax and feel at ease when discussing their personal problems.

Never allow your own personal beliefs or opinions to influence or prejudice your attitude and dealings towards the patient. Do not allow common media-portrayed stereotypes to cloud or affect your clinical judgement. Such patients are likely to pick up any negative cues or changes in behaviour that you may display. They are also likely to experience discrimination on a regular basis and would not expect their doctor to behave in a similar way.

Patients who experience prejudice simply request to be treated on an equal footing with any other person. Discriminatory behaviour of any sort is not befitting of a doctor and is not compatible with the GMC guidance on '*good medical practice*'. The doctor–patient relationship hinges on openness and mutual trust between the two parties for it to be successful. Prejudice and stereotyping is likely to damage this relationship beyond repair and must be avoided.

Index